I'M LOSING IT

AND MY GENES DON'T FIT

Weight Loss and Control Without Deprivation or Suffering

MARK STEINBERG PhD

Paperback ISBN: 979-8-9874856-4-4
Ebook ISBN: 979-8-9874856-5-1

Book design by Mayfly book design

Library of Congress Catalog Number: 2024923435
First Printing: 2024

Contents

PART I

A Heavy Burden

CHAPTER 1

For Starters

I Know This Is So

A s an astute observer, listener, and confidant to thousands, I can assert with complete conviction that most people find fault with their own appearance, and excess weight is an ongoing impediment to happiness. Body mass and body image are obsessive problems for tens of millions of Americans. Most of us are somewhat self-conscious about our bodies, dissatisfied with the way we look, and frustrated by how hard it is to lose weight.

You can trust me when I say this is so!

Less surprising is the alarming preponderance of obesity and associated health problems. And it's no wonder, given the plethora of available food (even at low prices especially for the less healthy food), the astute manufacturing, advertising, and manipulation by the food industry, plying us with salt, sugar, fat, and addictive foods, and the common genetic predisposition and human propensity to eat as much as we can (and store it).

Why do we eat so much? Because it's available, it gratifies, we are habituated, and there remains the "just in case of scarcity" genetic and emotional factors. Controlling our weight (and for most, that means losing some) is important, doable, and provides immense physical and psychological benefits.

I speak from personal experience, having struggled with weight most of my life. However, *I've lost over a hundred pounds* by following my own program, carefully synthesized through years of research, medical advice, experimentation, and gradual successful experience.

My weight battle began before I was born: a combination of genetics, cultural history, and environmental habits that I would eventually adopt from those around me. I refrain from blaming my parents. Loving and doting though they were, my Jewish parents endowed me with a good brain, a short stature, and a thick body, programmed to relish food and put on the pounds. Food and its rituals are central in Jewish culture (as in most cultures), and I was taught from an early age never to let smorgasbords or buffets make a profit from me!

The Yiddish term *fresser* means "one who eats a lot and enjoys food," in common parlance, a glutton, a pig). Yes, that was me. But I made many modifications in habits, appearance, taste, and attitude to achieve my success in losing weight. And I now proclaim that many of my genes just don't fit! My wardrobe and even my genetic manifestations are now altered!

Though genetics profoundly influence the development of many afflictions and diseases, they are not wholly deterministic. Each of us exerts significant influences on our health and other outcomes by our choices, habits, lifestyles, and the contributions from modern medicine. Through practice, determination, knowledge, and strategic planning, I have been able to preserve and develop much of the "good" genetic endowments and counteract some of the maladaptive ones, including the tendency to put on weight and carry forth my family history of obesity, diabetes, stroke, and heart disease. Through my adaptations, it turns out that some of my genes don't exactly fit who I have become!

Because most of us are so wrapped up in how we look, weight and appearance issues can easily take center stage and become battering rams that pummel our self-esteem and confidence. Millions suffer with anxiety, depression, despair, trauma, and shame—and weight and food issues, body image, and self-control can drive and reinforce these afflictions.

I want every person to feel good about themselves. Every single person has many likable qualities, notable accomplishments, affections, and positive feelings. Yet we often let obsessions or preoccupations about eating or body image "eat away" at the sense of self-worth. Our priority should be to feel positive about ourselves, whatever our food challenges happen to be. No more self-flagellation about willpower! None of us have sufficient willpower. Besides, willpower is not what reduces and manages weight.

Though I consider myself a very disciplined, careful, and well-organized person, I am self-indulgent, hedonistic, preoccupied with appetite and body, and tempted internally by conflicts and impulses about what I "deserve" versus the habits it takes to get the results that are ultimately more satisfying. Despite this lifelong battle, I am happy, enjoy good food regularly, accept my body and my limitations, and I am now more than 100 pounds lighter! In this book, I share the solutions I've found that made that possible and I examine the propelling forces we've all faced in the struggle to live peaceably with our bodies, minds, diets, and relationships with food.

Assorted factors related to our genetic precursors, physiological responses, environmental pressures, and habits collude to sabotage and defeat our efforts to be satisfied, disciplined, and healthy. So I do not profess to have a cure-all answer or sure-fire solution for every person, but I do have a systematic and successful weight-control regimen based on practicality and success. I will share how I personally lost lots of weight and continue to help many others lose weight and solve other related problems along the way—*without deprivation or suffering!*

Varying factors contribute to overeating and inappropriate eating that may seem to stack the deck against weight control and body/mind health, as well as self-image and confidence. Some of these factors may drive appetite and behavior for different individuals and at different times, and they may combine and shift. But by understanding some basic facts about human biology and our nutritional needs and eating habits, and by careful, gradual, and practical changes to eating, we can each comfortably control our weight and achieve a more satisfying relationship with our body, and with food.

CHAPTER 2

Good News That's New

I have good news to share about the challenge of losing and controlling weight. If you are hopeful and also skeptical, that's understandable. We've all read, heard, and tried a lot that hasn't panned out to the hype or the hope. What I refer to here is new information for most people that relates to health and weight reduction, even though the core principles governing our biology remain intact.

Much information is written about food contents, calories, nutritional values, recipes, diets, etc. Advising people to eat less (and less-fattening food) and exercise more is not new, and the boring repetition of the same is not helpful. As I promise to be *practical*, that translates to providing useful information that a person can act on, that is different from what has been tried, and that will result in the desired outcomes. As I focus on the newer stuff that can be a game changer for those wanting to get the upper hand on controlling their weight, I will include a review and some basic knowledge that's fundamental to weight successful loss.

Debunk willpower and determination in weight loss

I've often been advised that achieving goals requires "making a decision" that somehow precedes and facilitates digging in and persisting with steely determination. Such commitment is described in different ways using catchwords like "intention" and epithets like "God helps those who help themselves."

Such advice and "encouragement" has done *nothing* for me except adding to my guilt for not succeeding in the past, and lowering my motivation and confidence. Even disciplined and determined people get worn down, stressed, distracted, and unsuccessful at controlling their habits and bodies. Weight loss is not about willpower. It's about true understanding of how our bodies work and, with the correct information, taking charge of our habits and food intake in a manner that is *sustainable* and allows us to safely release unwanted pounds. This must be done without deprivation or suffering—or else it won't work and will be soon abandoned.

Sure, changing habits and preferences takes some effort and some *modest* sacrifice, but fortunately these are usually temporary. Planning and preparation, astute observation (keeping your eyes on the prize), and not being hard on yourself will pay much better dividends than a thankless redoubling of willpower.

Take charge of emotional influences on overeating and poor eating

We all know well that stress, adversity, and negative emotions trigger inappropriate eating (i.e., overeating, poor food choices, eating when not hungry). We have been advised repeatedly not to indulge in "emotional eating." But this advice does nothing to deter the impulses, drives, and habits that condition the brain and stomach to go to food for temporary emotional and physical relief from such discomfort.

Emotional eating is not about nutrition and satisfaction any more than a bucket is about repairing a leaky or burst pipe. At some point, we have to address and fix the source of the overflow. Rather than concentrate on thwarting the effect of emotional overwhelm (indiscriminate eating), I will explain and demonstrate how to regulate and gain control over runaway emotions so that eating habits become reformed gradually in a natural, satisfying, and productively fulfilling way.

Set yourself free from the strangling albatross of willpower

The idea of willpower implies control over and restraint of our impulses. Though each of us is ultimately responsible and accountable for what we do, control over impulses is highly attributable to physiology and its cumulative and pervasive influences on self-control.

As we shall see, willpower becomes a far less relevant aspect of self-control and restraint once physiology (biological regulation of blood sugar, appetite, satiety, and brain function) is regulated, normalized, and routinely managed.

This is not meant to exonerate choice and "free" will. But free will comes at the cost of being able to make conscious choices when we are not at the mercy of overpowering biological drives gone awry.

Understand food addictions and how to break them

A major factor in overeating is the effect that foods have on human biochemistry, which is reflected in appetite, blood chemistry, motivation, and compulsion. We tend to become strongly attracted (and sometimes addicted) to foods we eat habitually. We also tend to crave and gravitate toward foods that make us feel good—not necessarily healthy foods. The body and brain develop and exercise intuitive knowledge and motivation. But the sneaky reality for many is that food preferences and cravings (formed in response to the body's satiety from the foods it wants) actually cause unwanted and unhealthy reactions.

Sugar cravings are an easily understood example, but many other surreptitious processes by which people crave and eat foods make their bodies react poorly. Many of these foods may be "nutritious" but become toxic through overconsumption for some individuals. Many nutritious foods (eggs, whole grains, dairy, etc.) fall into these categories for some sensitive individuals, producing biochemical cravings for more along with diminishing satiety.

Beyond this unfortunate systemic response, the food industry has grown into a monolith of refined processing that conceals unhealthy amounts of sugar, salt, fat, and additives beneath the manufacture of tasty foods that are marketed to manipulate and attract our already-vulnerable and preconditioned appetites and behaviors. This perverted economic evolution warps our biological roots and results in poor diet, addictive eating, and rampant dissociation between the brain and gut centers of satiety and control. Simply put, the food we eat often causes and compels us to overeat more of the same.

The good news is that, by becoming aware of this dynamic and understanding the mechanisms, coupled with self-monitoring of cravings, eating patterns, and physiological reactions, we are better able to break food addictions. This is possible with fairly simple dietary changes that almost always result in healthier eating, less eating, and weight loss.

Use behavior modification to gradually change your habits

Behavior modification occurs constantly as we interact with our environment and respond to cues that strengthen or perpetuate the associations that reinforce our behaviors. Although many of our habit associations are not conscious and/or are manipulated by external forces (such as people's responses to us, marketing and advertising ploys, etc.), we need not be "victims" in the sense of being helplessly controlled (rather than suggestible). We can identify and deliberately alter our responses as well as change the triggers (cues) that tend to lock us into habits we may want to change. This holds true for forming new habits (preferably adaptive ones) and extinguishing maladaptive ones.

Though most people have some knowledge about behavior modification and perhaps even use some aspects of it, very few of us are equipped with the step-by-step practical implementation of these processes that are founded in the behavioral science application of learning theory. The principles of behavior modification, such as reinforcement, stimulus control, consequences, response cost, and reinforcement schedules, are critical elements of taking control of desired behavior change. One needn't be a behavioral scientist to employ these basic principles, but we do need to understand how they operate and see some pragmatic, plain-talk examples of how to use them to control our eating and our overall relationship with food.

I jokingly call this my version of CBT, but instead of "cognitive behavioral therapy," I mean *corpulent behavior therapy!* To observe, evaluate, and adjust our responses through structured alterations in line with principles and schedules of reinforcement and extinction are far more effective than trying to change our behavior by trying to change or reframe our thoughts. I help my patients use statistically reliable methods of probability, frequency, intensity, and duration to end addictions and reduce unwanted behaviors while building adaptive ones at the same time. Within these pages, I share some of these valuable techniques.[1]

Use a powerful treatment to get rid of self-sabotage

We all do things at times that are counter to our best interests and even our intent. Such self-sabotage is sneaky, often not conscious, and perplexing to overcome. In my decades of work with people's thoughts, motivations, and histories, I've abandoned fanciful psychological theories about subconscious influences, childhood programming, furtive death wishes, and unconscious "undeserving" attitudes in favor of a scientifically proven, practical, and rapid way to defeat self-sabotage. This quick and effective technique that is fundamental to Thought Field Therapy (TFT) is a treatment for *psychological reversal*—when a person's thoughts and action are in direct conflict with their goals. Appropriately applied neurological finger tapping, targeted to negative thought fields that self-sabotage, clears the way toward unobstructed follow through with one's actual intentions and desires.

Voice Technology, which is the most advanced application of Thought Field Therapy, eliminates negative emotions, stress, intrusive thinking, shame, fear of failure, and other problems within minutes. The technique is instrumental in correcting self-sabotage that interferes with motivation and successful behavior change. I often do this technique by phone with my patients, so they have constant and immediate access to my assistance when needed. I also teach self-help techniques.

Getting rid of self-sabotage regularly assists greatly in attaining better self-control of emotions, behaviors, and food intake.

---

1. This topic is outlined in greater depth in my book, *Life Control: Take Charge and Get Ahead.*

Improve your sleep and boost your metabolism naturally

Training the brain with EEG neurofeedback improves overall brain health and makes a person mentally stronger, more durable, more flexible, and more resilient. This method has proven effective for a vast majority of patients. Along with relieving anxiety, depression, trauma, and other negative emotions, neurofeedback reduces stress and improves sleep—two major factors in controlling appetite and weight.

The "in tune" harmony of neurofeedback increases calmness and patience and modulates appetite and satiety by making your brain more aware of your body. Because mindless eating goes hand in hand with dissociation between emotions and physiological satiety, eating yourself into self-loathing or "food stupor" is less likely when your brain is in tune with your body awareness.

Change taste and appetite from fatty junk foods to healthy slimming foods

You may be challenged by longstanding habits and tastes that make you crave and reach for calorie dense and fattening foods; you may have been eating such foods for decades and wonder how you can change. But believe me: you can change what appeals to your taste buds. Such adaptation is usually gradual, does not require deprivation, and is facilitated as you substitute healthier, natural, unprocessed foods into your diet. You'll be surprised how satisfied and full you feel without the bloated stuffed sensation induced by fatty and chemicalized foods. You also feel full for longer periods as your body adapts to healthier fare.

Though you can still indulge in your favorite go-to foods, you'll tend to do so far less often—and, as you eat them less frequently, your tastes will naturally undergo change. Imagine craving the foods that are the healthiest! That can happen! As you *gradually* transition your diet, you will find that you actually prefer healthy food more than fatty junk food.

Use exercise as an assist, rather than a requirement for weight loss

In youth, we can get away with a lot of poor choices—in food and lots of other areas. Our metabolism is faster, our muscles and blood vessels more elastic, and recovery is generally quicker. As we age, these functions and organs slow and degrade. Capacity for exercise decreases (fitness level adjusted notwithstanding), recovery from injury and exertion takes longer, metabolism slows, and our bodies thicken. Though exercise is very important throughout life, we cannot rely on workouts to maintain weight and/or prevent obesity.

Physical movement is crucial to facilitate faster metabolism, reduce stress, and improve circulation, sleep, and overall well-being. Many people have mobility limits, physical impairments, or injuries that limit exercise. Though quite important, exercise plays less of a role in weight reduction than proper eating and metabolism balance. Moving just a bit more on a regular basis (within one's physical limits) helps tremendously. Start with small steps to increase movement and/or exercise by 10 percent every two weeks. If you can walk ten blocks, try stretching it to eleven. Aim for what is known as a JND (just noticeable difference) in effort and tolerance. You'll be surprised to feel how your tolerance, mobility, and fitness improve little by little.

More good news is that you don't have to burn (or count) calories to counter your appetite. You can use exercise as an assist in an overall program that will modify how you eat, look, and what you weigh. Think of what an electric bike does: you still have to pedal, but the motorized assist provides a boost for hills, momentum, and the pleasure of riding without drudgery.

Modest and consistent exercise will similarly help you stay motivated, enjoy movement, revert it to a habit, and provide your body with the necessary stimulation to function and process food more efficiently.

Be aware of the development and efficacy of new medications

Many weight-loss strategies include drugs to suppress appetite. Among these were amphetamine variations that have many serious and deleterious side effects. They suppress appetite, but they also are highly addictive and destructive to organs, most notably the heart. Amphetamines are also *very bad* for the brain.

Fortunately, a revolution in the pharmacology of blood sugar and appetite has occurred and continues to evolve. A new class of medications that was developed originally to lower and control blood sugar in people with diabetes, a progressive and devastating disease for many millions of Americans, whose incidence is sharply increasing. These newer medications also facilitate appetite suppression and weight loss—and they can actually be good for the heart. Cumulative studies indicate that for those with cardiovascular risk factors, these medications reduce the incidence and risk of cardiac events and strokes.

Control blood sugar

Intricate and delicate biological mechanisms signal and regulate our brain, endocrine system, and organs in order to supply and control the flow of nutrients to our cells. These mechanisms release and store energy and promote the growth and health of cells as well as excrete waste and toxins. A fundamental part of this process is the management of blood sugar.

Our blood sugar level and concentration (glycemia) is a measure of the amount of glucose in our blood. Unregulated blood sugar levels lead to many serious health issues, especially diabetes. If we eat too much food with sugar (and carbohydrates that the body converts to sugar), we can develop *insulin resistance*, meaning the cells in your muscles, fat, and liver cannot easily absorb the glucose from your blood. The pancreas then makes more insulin to help glucose enter the cells. Over time, the body does not respond as well to the insulin, and our blood sugar rises to unhealthy levels. Swings in our blood sugar can invoke desperate hunger pangs and extreme fluctuations in energy. Eating food with high sugar content gives a quick spike in blood sugar, energy, and satiety, only to quickly rebound in a rollercoaster drop in the aforementioned.

Basically, our body management of blood sugar is intimately tied to how we feel—our energy, appetite, satiety, concentration, and mood. Low blood sugar makes misery; high blood sugar results in disease.

If blood sugar could talk, it might say:

"I respond to what you regul'ate."

"If we go steady, I'll be faithful and help you."

"When you overload me, you'll feel bad later."

"We can be intimate without being too sweet."

"I don't like feast or famine."

Consider the example of building and sustaining a fire: Since paper ignites easily, lighting it will quickly yield a substantial flame. However, it burns quickly and is unlikely able to ignite other fuel for a lasting flame. Kindling wood is typically used to start a controlled fire; it is pretty easily ignited, and twigs tend to burn longer than paper. However, unless it burns long enough to ignite logs, the fire will extinguish. Heavier logs will sustain fire the longest, but it's more difficult to get them to ignite. So a combination of easily ignited material with longer-burning wood is needed to build and sustain a fire.

Sweets, such as confections, ice cream, soda, etc., are like paper fuel—they give a quick burst of energy, but rapidly fizzle out, plummeting blood sugar levels. Carbohydrates—bread, pasta, chips, rice, and many ingredients in processed foods—are like kindling. They burn longer than paper (e.g., the concentrated sugar example), but soon expire their energy, returning blood sugar to much lower levels.

The logs of nutrition are good quality protein and fat, along with slower metabolizing carbohydrates found in vegetables, legumes, and some fruits (whole). These should be the dietary mainstay for consistent energy and controlling and regulating healthy blood sugar levels that moderate appetite and food consumption. Great practical news is that by gaining dominion over your blood sugar, you will find tremendous advantage over controlling your appetite, food behaviors, weight, appearance, and health.

Focus on the good news

Indeed, it is profoundly good news that weight control and food relationships can be accomplished without deprivation, suffering, or yielding to the merciless burden of willpower. Though it's most important to concentrate on and utilize the good news, it's also important to be cognizant of the bad news about nature's (including our human nature) challenges.

Read on you see how to use this knowledge to empower your efforts and achieve greater success and peace.

CHAPTER 3

Bad News
You Already Know

A dhering to my promise to be encouraging and practical without resorting to platitudes or trite advice and lectures, I aim to deliver *reminders* about the nature and biology we are up against. My purpose is not to nag, scare, or even motivate you by listing the many disadvantages of eating poorly and being overweight. You already know those.

Instead, I want you to review the bad news with a mind toward congratulating yourself! That's right—congratulate yourself that you are taking on a significant and gargantuan task of battling and counteracting the natural and environmental forces that *conspire* to make you fat and less healthy. The universe may not be consciously out to get you personally, but it seems that its many natural principles and operations often deflate and defeat even the most noble and persistent efforts to battle deleterious effects. Therefore, let's start with an attitude of stoic determination and self-encouragement as we try to be heroes in this difficult undertaking.

The main adversaries are time and nature. Our bodies naturally wear down and become less resilient, efficient, and able to tolerate and metabolize excess. Other challenges include our tendencies to be self-indulgent, cater to impulses and appetites, and the vast complex of industrial manufacturing, advertising, and manipulation that hijacks and corrupts normal eating and nutrition for humans.

Disease and Declining Health

In light of the many biological and environmental forces that can negatively impact us, it's remarkable how the human body withstands invasion, repairs itself, and often flourishes. Each of us has a limited time on this planet, the course of that trajectory plotted by genetic factors, lifestyle choices and habits, environment, happenstance, and—if our beliefs incline such acceptance—divine providence or fate.

We can take many steps to influence and improve our health and our body capacities. Yet many of the outcomes are heavily determined by genetics. We are constantly grappling with nature and, as you have probably discovered, nature eventually wins. Mortality aside (let's be cheerful about reality and the time we have), we can do a lot to make life longer and certainly more fruitful and enjoyable.

From birth on, we develop with predictable, if not exact or uniform, changes as our cells trigger, mature, and die. In our formative years, we gain strength and physical capabilities along with brain growth that facilitates survival. As this process occurs, it takes time to integrate curiosity, risk-taking, and fear modulation with a natural puerile sense of invincibility. We cut our teeth on life's intrusions, traumas, and lessons. Usually and hopefully, we learn caution, wisdom, and self-control—our allies in making peace with nature. For a time, we can work with nature and even fool or delay nature's edicts. But the inevitability of aging and decline lurks and stalks even the most robust, stalwart, and lucky.

Hormonal and hair changes take their toll, as do the efficiency and time needed to heal as we age. Injuries accumulate, and structural suppleness and flexibility diminish. Arthritis is common. Skin sags and wrinkles. We lose muscle mass and tone. Eyesight and hearing eventually weaken. Metabolism slows down, and bodies thicken.

All of this is normal, as natural as trees growing and shedding leaves. Besides the inevitable and expected wearing out of our bodies, we have accidents and traumas. Genetic anomalies may cause debilitation and even curtail lifespan. We are subject to many diseases and degenerative conditions. It is also increasingly apparent that diet contributes significantly to diseases and longevity.

Diets Don't Work

We know of so many angles to proper diets, healthy nutrition, and methods to lose weight. Your interest in this book implies that you have investigated and perhaps tried numerous different ways of eating. There are supplements galore, supposed "genius hacks" based on scientific and nutritional principles, "special" natural weight-loss foods, and legions of recommendations about when, what, and how to eat—each touting their own "proven" efficacy, usually with promises of rapid weight loss without pain.

Skeptical? You are wise to be. Disappointed with the methods you've tried? (Tell me about it.) You are not alone in your disillusionment. The simple truth is that diets rarely work. You may shed pounds at first (often water weight), only to find them return. Most weight-loss diets and schemes are unsustainable. And many are unhealthy or dangerous. Short-term gains (in success) and losses (in pounds) are almost always replaced by eventual gains (in pounds) and losses (in motivation and health).

Amid the controversy about proper eating, good nutrition, and effective eating for health, satiety, and weight loss, there is little for the hapless consumer to rely on. Perhaps the safest consensus is the advice to cut down on processed foods and eat lots of fresh vegetables. Good advice . . . and good luck.

There is no magic diet. Different eating patterns work for different people and may vary according to ethnic heritage and where you live. They may also change over time according to your body's changes and status.

Appearance and Clothes

Attention to appearance varies greatly among individuals. Some are fastidious and/or fashion conscious while others put little stock in trends and fashion, preferring simplicity and economy in their utilitarian approach to garb. Suffice it to say that whatever you wear, when it no longer fits, you become concerned. That might be an understatement. When clothes become snug or unwearable, we may panic and even mount self-hatred. We

17

gaze in the closet with dismay and in the mirror with degrees of confusion, disgust, and loathing. How could this happen?

Decades ago, I had a very talented tailor upon whom I relied regularly and increasingly to let out the waist on my pants. He was diplomatic enough to rarely comment; but when he did, he smiled and said he was happy that I was enjoying "the good life." This was little consolation for the polite interpretation that prosperity was undergirding my increasing girth. While there is truth to the idea that increased income may correspond with richer or tastier food habits, it's nonetheless the reality that healthy, natural food is more expensive than cheaper processed food. Poverty is a gateway to poor diet, weight gain, and disease.

It's been years since those days when I abashedly and regularly visited the tailor to let out my pants. Recently, I've renewed my relationship with a current tailor whom I've paid thousands of dollars to *take in* the fabrics of my extensive wardrobe (shirts and suits included). This time around, it's a proud delight.

I've always been interested in clothes, style, and dressing carefully. Nothing off the shelf fits me, as I am five foot six and have short arms. But, as I like to say, "Tailors are less expensive than orthopedic surgeons."

Fitting into clothes or buying new ones can be a powerful motivator for regimes and disciplines to get in shape. It can also work the other way around, contributing to frustration, shame, and hopelessness. Rare is the person who can still fit into their high school clothes. We do our best and move on.

I cling to the motto, "Do your best, look your best, be your best." It's a high and worthy aspiration, leaping ahead of the realities of hard work, change, and much failure along the way.

Self-Confidence and Self-Esteem

The obvious corollary to weight gain is an accompanying loss of confidence and perhaps a plummet in self-esteem. So much of our identity is tied up in how we look. There is also much social shaming and thoughtless commentary about being fat.

It doesn't work to ignore obesity, nor to pretend we are not bothered by less-than-flattering appearance. We may endure periods of "The heck with it; I tried my best. I guess I'll just be large." We may feel sorry for ourselves. But eventually, it's time to try again with renewed hope and strategy.

It takes courage, maturity, faith, wisdom, knowledge, and planning to navigate the tricky terrain of balancing discipline and self-control with self-acceptance and an identity not solely tied to appearance.

Long ago, I developed a definition of self-esteem: self-esteem is a composite of *What am I good at?* And *What am I good for?* The *good at* comprises skills and competencies. The *good for* is based upon a sense of being loved and valued, worthy and needed, and it must be unconditional to be real.

These descriptions still hold up usefully and I adhere to them for myself and others, regardless of how anyone looks.

Harder to Move

Another difficult reality that's part of the bad news is that, as we age and/or gain weight, movement becomes more difficult. The orthopedic doctors say that every extra pound on our body is equivalent to five extra pounds on our knees.

A cruel irony is that being heavy makes it harder to move, and less movement makes us heavier: a terribly vicious cycle. Whether through injuries, physical limitations, and/or the burden of obesity, many people find movement (or any exercise) too strenuous, taxing, and unpleasant.

Yet movement itself—any physical movement—has many benefits for physical and mental health. Even minor increases in movement reduce stress, boost metabolism, can reduce or allay hunger, and help hormonal flow, sleep, and self-regulation.

Physical movement should and can be a joy. You don't have to be an athlete or love exercise. In fact, as we age past thirty, exercise becomes much less effective as a means of losing weight (though it can help control weight and should be done as regularly as one can for many other health, hobby, and happiness reasons).

Humans are not designed to be sedentary. But our modern lifestyles promote and reinforce way too much sedentariness. I've heard it said, "Sitting is the new smoking."

As a veteran psychologist steeped in the science of habit change, I have long practiced and recommended incremental steps to shape new and adaptive behaviors. I suggest the *ten percent strategy*: Start where you can with movement and increase by 10 percent each week. If you can do ten sit-ups, graduate to eleven. This increase is well under the threshold of what we call a just noticeable difference (JND). Your body won't notice the difference, and your mind will tolerate it. If you can walk five blocks at first, try walking five-and-a-half blocks the week after. Pretty soon (but not overdoing or rushing it) you will double your capacity. Moreover, you will form a new habit that is easier to sustain. Who knows? You may even begin to look forward to your walks.

CHAPTER 4

The Plot Thickens

Metabolism, Muscles, Gravity, Chemistry

I love and hate the saying, "Gravity doesn't care." I love it because it's a stark reminder that natural forces aren't personal. If the universe is out to get me, it will also get the rest of us too. Reality is better to contend with than to ignore. If there ever is equality, natural forces are its embodiment. I hate that gravity doesn't care, because there's no arguing with it!

What this foray into philosophy means for us physically is that, even when we carefully obey the laws of gravity, its gradual effects on our bodies make appearance sag (organs inside too), endurance flag, and movement harder. Gravity is an ever-present and easily noticeable reminder of a host of natural processes that wear us down as we age.

Metabolism slows as we get older, taking steeper declines after age thirty. Slower metabolism means we need less food, because we burn calories at a slower rate. This contributes significantly to weight gain. Hormones change and, along with metabolic slowing, our internal chemistry becomes less efficient at burning unnecessary calories.

As we age, muscle mass decreases and more of it turns to fat. We simply can't eat the amounts we used to (our bodies don't need as much food). We are also more sensitive to toxins and excesses, even occasionally (think alcohol and the potentially devastating impact of stimulant drugs or depressants on the heart and lungs). Our body composition changes, making outward tone less taut and defined, and the visceral fat around our organs accumulates.

The factors of age-related slowdown, progression of and debilitation by injuries or illness, the reduced effectiveness of vigorous exercise to counter caloric intake, and the intruding and compelling forces of manufactured and processed food, along with our evolutionary predisposition to seek and store food all combine as some natural conspiracy to make weight control quite the challenge.

Thickening With Age

Although some individuals are stocky, squat, roly-poly, or overweight from a young age, the vast majority are much narrower in youth than we are later. Peruse pictures of yourself, and you'll be amazed at how you've "filled out," regardless of how much weight you've put on.

Look at photos of celebrities and others, and you'll see the same phenomenon. It's most apparent in the face. Jowls and neck become thicker, and the whole face is wider as time passes. Even those who have "work done" (plastic surgery) cannot hide the relentless effects of aging. Bodies widen even more. It's difficult to accept this unflattering reality.

How and why does this happen? For reasons described in the Bad News chapter, our bodies change with natural age progression. Hormonal and metabolic changes cause us to thicken. Even those who maintain weight within a healthy range show unmistakable signs of widening. It's just part of getting older.

We look wistfully at yesteryear's pictures of ourselves and regretfully pine, *How did I get to look like this*? Keeping in good shape, maintaining good habits and hygiene, caring for appearance through wardrobe and makeup, and perhaps cosmetic enhancements can help. Yet age makes us different and more-mature versions of ourselves. Let's be thankful that we get there, despite wishing for the lankiness we may have once had. You may have been skinnier decades ago—but you were also most certainly less wise.

The wise step we can take is to limit or reverse weight gain and counteract the many deleterious effects of aging that come with the territory of more birthdays.

Fat Kids

I really feel sorry for fat kids. I don't look down on them, nor do I blame or shame them. As a psychologist concerned with human development, and working with children and families for many decades, I deal with many aspects of childhood wellness and problems. I understand the developmental challenges many children face, and I treat them professionally to maximize normalization and potential to live a happy and productive life.

I'm not a nutrition expert, nor do I hyperfocus on diet to police the intake of kids. However, we do have to face the reality that diet has a major impact on mental functioning as well as physical health, along with the fact that childhood obesity has become epidemic. Fast and junk food pervade the diets of a majority of children. Besides impairing their attention and behavior, sugar makes people addicted and fat while on the way to bringing many diseases.

We have long noted and measured the pernicious effects of poor or neglectful parenting, childhood trauma, academic difficulties, and social ostracism on later development and functioning. With proper intervention and support, many developmental challenges can be surmounted. Most of us have overcome obstacles that stalled us earlier in life. Good upbringing, environmental supports, and healthy emotional environments go a long way to combat disadvantages and enable us to meet challenges.

Yet we see that early successes in life are fundamental to establishing a grounded and resilient identity along with self-confidence and good self-esteem. In the domain of controlling our body and weight, early developmental health and success is crucial to making the adaptations required as we age. The supple and energetic school athlete will face the metabolic and maturational challenges common to everyone, but a history of fitness and discipline in youth predicts and paves the path for better adjustments as age progresses.

Fat kids don't have this preparedness. Their history, experiences, and memories deviate markedly from growing up with competence, agility, inclusion, and social validation. They don't have a history of fitness, energy, and healthy habits to remember, build upon, and restore. Childhood obesity—besides all its physical and social drawbacks—prevents children from calling upon a developmental foundation for proper eating and self-care. They inherit a handicap, genetic and environmental, thrusting them into the game of life where most everyone else has already scored more points. For fat kids, catching up later is ever more difficult. Yet it can and must be done.

Genes: Do Yours Fit?

The title, *My Genes Don't Fit,* is a wry commentary on my own conflicts and battles over time with myself: who I am, who and what I want to be, and the preprogramming and limitations imposed by genetics.

Though not entirely deterministic, genetic predisposition extrudes throughout development and heavily influences many life outcomes. The role and power of choice notwithstanding (and I am a staunch proponent of choice and personal responsibility, even having written books about it), many outcomes are beyond our control. I will never be able to dunk a basketball (darn it!), run a four-minute mile, or give birth. Each of us is born with a gender, an ethnicity, and a rich genetic heritage that includes strengths and weaknesses of many kinds.

Reviewing my own development in light of my genetics, I see that many characteristics seem to fit, whereas other seem foreign to the way I view myself and my aspirations. I appreciate being smart and being part of a genetic pattern that shows robustness and relative longevity. I don't like my short and stocky stature, the disease factors that run in my family (heart disease, diabetes, depression, allergies, schizophrenia). I deplore the "personality" predispositions I inherited, which I also take reluctant ownership of, such as an indulgent leaning toward sarcasm, criticism, and negativity.

To the extent that I can consciously choose, develop character and integrity, and cannily work with the clay I am given, I am living in ways that defy many genetic predictions and influences. As a recipient of grace and mercy, I follow a spiritual path that provides discipline, humility, and forgiveness. Through heart surgery, I have a new lease on life. I've managed to avoid (or at least forestall) the diabetes that runs in my family and took my mother's legs before ending her life. I've overcome my own dark days of despair and mental illness and have been blessed with a long career helping others.

And I've *lost over a hundred pounds* while coming to terms with repairing, accepting, and loving my body, as well as developing a fair and rewarding relationship with food and eating. In so many ways, I no longer suffer!

So now some of my genes don't fit who I've become. And the "jeans" that fit are the ones I've bought since losing lots of weight. *Hallelujah!*

What about you? Are tight jeans making you miserable? Are your blood genes holding you back? Let's do something useful and wonderful about both.

Remember—and I will keep reminding you—this is a practical book about developing a bountiful love for yourself, improving your confidence and self-acceptance, working out a reasonable and sustainable relationship and habits with yourself and food, and shedding some pounds so you feel better, look better, and enjoy more health and fewer limits.

Reality is manageable, though at times difficult and overwhelming. We need to keep our eyes on the prize while acknowledging and navigating the many daunting obstacles that arise.

You are commended for surviving, continuing to try, for your intelligence, integrity, and faith. You are affirmed for who you are beneath the skin-deep beauty to which we unrealistically aspire and compare ourselves.

My pep talk is sincere and hopefully motivating. Belief should be earned and informed by both good and bad news. There's more of both types to come.

CHAPTER 5

Everybody Loves Some Body

My mother was five feet, two inches tall. She was a powerhouse in many ways. Her love, generosity, and empathy knew no bounds. She would give you the shirt off her back (and given her dimensions, it would likely be too wide and too short). She was a professional educator and, later in life, a painter and sculptor. She had a keen and unbridled interest in people and in doing good.

As far as I can remember, my mom was always overweight. She stopped cigarette smoking in her later years, but the damage clearly had been done. She was an advanced diabetic who suffered a debilitating stroke and had both legs amputated. Toward the end of her life, she suffered severe dementia and was fed through a tube.

During her long career, she taught Home Economics to high school students and served as a vice principal. For a time, she was also the chief dietician at Greenpoint Hospital in Brooklyn. Ever the Jewish mother, traditional in her culture and practices, she was guided by kosher rules and informed by the nutritional advice of her time. This included lots of kosher meat; thus I was fed "only the best kosher steaks money could buy." Unfortunately, I also supplemented this part of my diet with processed food containing lots of fat. Genes, my mother's cooking, and my indulgent and voracious appetite helped me become a *fresser*. I take responsibility for my part in loving food and eating too much of it.

I loved food and unfortunately let this become a worship. Outside of my kosher home, I furtively sought and welcomed opportunities to eat "forbidden" (nonkosher) foods. I preferred my friend's mother's cheap hot dogs to my mom's expensive steaks, and the occasions that led me to ham sandwiches or sausage, which I coveted salaciously as if it were *food pornography*. In addition to sugar, I couldn't get enough of the processed foods high in salt, fat, and preservatives. Sodium and nitrites snuck inevitably into my diet.

Christian writer C. S. Lewis joked about his "lusting for breakfast." Such was my vice.

Due to a speedy metabolism and a fanatical interest in sports, I exercised rigorously up until my late twenties. Thus I was able to burn off excess energy and avoid obesity until my thirties. During adolescence, I developed an interest (and later a fetish) in natural foods. I learned to cook, enjoyed it, and for years I cut down on junk food and ate whole fresh foods. Adult life, temptation, and sloppy habits gradually caught up with me, and I steadily put on the pounds.

What a Figure!

My mother didn't like being short and pudgy; but apparently, she failed to modify her diet and habits. One of her favorite stories that she told many times was about her envy/jealousy of her classmate, Bess Myerson.

Bess Myerson was the first Jewish Miss America, a politician, actress, and model. My mother often reminisced enviously about how fabulous Bessie looked in a bathing suit. Clearly, my mother envied and adored Bessie. My mother wanted so badly to be gorgeous too.

A relatively small percentage of people are blessed with outstanding looks (according to relative cultural standards). Even fewer have and retain hourglass shapes or six-pack abs with flattering hips and proportions. Truth be told, most of us look in the mirror and wish an idealized someone else looked back at us. It's hard to get over this. We are naturally given to pride, envy, covetousness, and self-pity. Then the world piles it on.

I'm not suggesting we are helpless. But it does take determination, struggle, and maturity to accept and appreciate who you are: the special and unique creation that God saw fit to bring forth with all your selfish preoccupations, gnawing appetites, and accumulating adiposity.

Everybody loves some body: usually *somebody else's*. Admiration is one thing; but envy can tear you apart.

A lilting love song was recorded and made famous decades ago by Dean Martin, "Everybody Loves Somebody" by songwriters, Irving Taylor / Ken Lane. This well-known song is about romantic love of a highly desirable, sought-after partner. Happiness comes through finding and adoring the perfect one. Such fantasized adulation can also take the form of jealous projection.

Here is my version (with substituted lyrics):

Everybody Loves Some Body

Everybody loves some body sometime
Everybody envies someone else
Something in your figure tells me
I really should tighten my belt.

Everybody finds somebody someplace
Looking better than they think they do
Your appearance has just told me
I'll never look as good as you.

If I had it in my power
I'd arrange for my shape to be more thin
Then every minute, every hour.
I'd delight in the body that I'm in.

Everybody loves some body sometime
Why am I just plain and grow so fat?
I long for a body that is sublime
A figure people can't stop looking at.

Everybody loves some body sometime
Others seem to have beauty I lack
Maybe if I could love myself more
Many people would love me back.

Your body may not be the one you want. Work on enjoying and improving the one you have. Pulchritude beckons with attraction and temptation, but it's fleeting and highly overrated. It's far better to admire beauty as an art form and with well-wishing for those endowed.

Bess Myerson was ravishing in a swimsuit. Beyond the ephemeral limelight, her life was fraught with misery: criminal convictions, divorce, cancer, stroke, and dementia.

My mother was short, dumpy, and she gorged with abandon. But, *oh my*, was she ever beautiful!

PART II

Obesity: Disease or Disorder?

CHAPTER 6

Is Obesity a Disease?

As the general issue of weight control draws increasing attention, greater credence is being given to the belief that obesity is a disease. Moreover in some medical circles, it is also assumed to be a brain disease. This thinking blends the scientific disciplines of metabolism, gastroenterology, and neuroscience with social and behavioral science. Calling obesity a disease (particularly a brain disease) can affect how people regard themselves and their beliefs and actions about their "choices" and "willpower."

My background and practice in clinical neuropsychology, buttressed by a longstanding interest in the role of food and diet in mental health, along with my personal saga of weight issues, makes me keenly interested in and fairly opinionated regarding this turnabout in classification and assumptions.

What Is a Disease?

"Disease" is defined as a particular abnormal condition that adversely affects the structure or function of all or part of an organism and is not immediately due to an external injury. Diseases are assumed to be medical conditions which have known causes and distinctive groups of symptoms, signs, or anatomical changes.

The presence of disease indicates abnormality. This implies the need to remove contaminating foreign bodies or corrupting agents. Presumably, disease will not abate without proper medical treatment; diseases require *cures*. With this model, patients are relatively helpless to overcome disease without medical intervention.

We can all agree that cancer is a disease. Parkinson's is a disease, as are heart abnormalities and infections such as COVID. Alternatively, many conditions and deviations from normality are known as *disorders*. A disorder is a *disruption* in regular body structure or function. As the term suggests, it is a lack or absence of *order*.

Attention-deficit is called attention-deficit disorder. We have also labeled learning and behavior disorders. In mental health, we have anxiety disorders, depressive disorders, adjustment disorders, etc.

Disorder is a more fitting concept for many ailments and afflictions, because it encompasses the relationship—often intermittent, transitional, or shifting—between normality and abnormality. They are related and recognized in terms of each other and the prevailing dominance of *order* or *disorder*. The difference between order and disorder is the degree and consistency of the organization and stabilization of our *internal default states*.

A default state (also called default network mode) is the pattern of neural network firing that our brain does internally when it reverts to its familiar resting mode. Default states can be normal, in the sense of flexible and healthy, or familiar but dysregulated, in the sense that, due to habit, the brain acts as if dysregulation is the normal default mode. Order deteriorates into disorder when our default states are disorganized and lack coherent feedback and integration, thereby inducing or maintaining dysfunctional patterns. For example, a mood disorder reflects the brain's difficulty and instability at regulating mood flows, variations in arousal, and resilience. Similarly, a sleep disorder occurs when one cannot routinely transition among necessary states of arousal to enter and maintain sleep stages.

Why Does This Matter?

The medical establishment has classified alcoholism and obesity as diseases. Why not just accept it and let it be judged as such? Because it matters for the characteristics described above: namely, if it's a disease, it must be treated with the conventional tools of medicine. Not doing so would deny and deprive patients of "necessary" treatments to eradicate physical causes and abnormalities, making symptoms persist and health decline.

If obesity is a disease, then those afflicted may tend to deny responsibility for its origin and continuation. With the disease model, obese people may feel exonerated from behaviors and health practices that contributed to the condition. Their health and fate are in the hands and plans of physicians who attempt to eliminate the disease through drugs or surgery, perhaps "relieving" them of their own duties regarding their "cure" except for compliance with the medical regimen.

Even with a disease model for alcoholism and drug addiction, doctors and treatment facilities recommend or include collateral interventions aimed at reforming patient lifestyles and behaviors. Such interventions may be very helpful. But the bottom line is that "therapies" and meetings cannot substitute for treating the afflicted organ. Cancer support groups may be useful, but they don't treat the cancer. Collateral treatments that improve attitude may assist the healing process, but the afflicted organs still require biological treatment.

The issues of etiology and persistence of conditions such as obesity, addictions, and mental illnesses are complicated by murky crossovers between scientific evidence and theories about the cause-and-effect relationships between behaviors and organic health. An example of contradictory belief and practice is easily demonstrated in the conventional approach to anxiety and depression. For these conditions, mainstream medicine will typically recommend medication.

Mood disorders are assumed to be due to neurotransmitter deficiencies, so the appropriate solution is deemed chemical. However, physicians may also recommend psychotherapy (talking about it). In my view, this is hypocritical lip service. Here's why: if the problem is only neurochemical, then why would talking about it about it address the physiological problem? In what way is that a solution? Conversely, if some form of talk therapy solves or reverses anxiety or depression, then why flood the body with harsh chemicals having known adverse side effects and dependencies?

Pediatricians often prescribe medications (particularly dangerous stimulants) to children with attention-deficit disorder based upon an assumption that without medicinally straightening out their neurotransmitters, they cannot learn or behave properly. Yet there is also a parallel thrust for parenting skills, behavioral interventions, and academic and lifestyle modifications. In theory, these interventions would complement and augment each other. Confusion derives from what you believe is the actual cause and its logical requirement for a lock-and-key solution. It is disingenuous to have it both ways. Either the meds fix it and external interventions are superfluous, or the environmental solutions are critical, thus deflating the purported organic disease model as causal.

Certainly I endorse good parenting, behavior modification, healthy diet, and appropriate educational services. I've built my career around these cornerstones. In some situations, as temporary relief or for crisis management, psychotropic medications may be helpful. And collateral interventions can by synergistic. If you contend that the problem is primarily neurochemical and organic, then you may discount the central solution as environmental and behavioral. With conviction that social influences, behavioral conditioning, and characterological forces are what constitute the problem, then you will not look to chemical solutions as necessary or even appropriate.

What About Brain Disease?

With the contemporary thinking that asserts that alcoholism, addictions, and obesity are brain diseases, those afflicted with these problems may infer and believe that they cannot control their behaviors constellating around indulgence, habit, cravings, and relapses. The difficulties and self-fulfilling prophecies deduced from such a position are obvious and unavoidable.

"I cannot control my appetites, cravings, and behaviors."

"There's something wrong with my brain that I cannot fix."

"I should not be punished or even held responsible for the damage I cause to myself or others."

"Critics and natural consequences victimize me and induce shame and guilt I don't deserve."

After years of struggling with weight, self-control, addictions, and the attendant guilt and shame, patients are eager to latch on to explanations and diagnoses that absolve them from personal and societal blame. Though understandable, such pronouncements may also hinder personal responsibility.

I have been an addict, and my own son died from drug addiction. I treat addictions and their associated and underlying conditions (known as comorbidities). I am empathetic and sympathetic to the terrible conundrums of those caught in the grip of these maladies.

I have no doubt in my mind—nor in the medical evidence—that poor diet, overuse of alcohol, and addictive drugs cause and result in diseases, including brain diseases.

But here's some breaking news: behaviors are not diseases!

Cirrhosis of the liver is a deadly disease, and chronic alcohol excess causes it. Diabetes is a devastating disease, and sugar causes it. But heavy drinking itself and eating too much cake are not diseases. They are compulsions and habits caused by the interactions of these unhealthy substances with the dysregulation of the majority of Americans who have metabolic disorders. Metabolic disorders are frequently the normal consequences of abnormal and dysregulated eating and nutrition.

When the vicious cycle of ingestion and indulgence, relief and withdrawal, craving and repetition reaches its predictable unhealthy outcomes, we should not fault the body for reacting as it's supposed to. A nutritional expert and colleague has likened this to "blaming the fire department when it shows up to put out the fire."

Diagnosis By Prescription

Sometimes physicians will "confirm" a hypothesized diagnosis by pointing to the patient's response to a medication. Thus if a rowdy or inattentive child focuses better on a stimulant, then this is presumed evidence of attention-deficit disorder. This seeming empirical justification short-cuts the differential diagnostic process and conflates effect with cause in an unscientific manner.

Patients about to undergo surgery are routinely given a dose of anxiolytics (anxiety medication) right before surgery to calm and prepare them. Obviously, the expected and observed response is a significant general relaxation, even a mild "high." We certainly should not pull this response out of context to conclude that the patient has an anxiety disorder!

Yet this seat-of-the-pants approach is used to assess and make diagnostic conclusions about other state-related disorders. *Let's prescribe an antidepressant and, if the patient feels better, we'll know they have depression.*

Let's not overlook two common scenarios that undercut this hypothesis. First, many obviously and historically depressed people do not respond well to antidepressants; but they are clearly depressed. Second, it's common in medical practice to try numerous medications in combination or consecutively when patients don't respond adequately to the first medication. Diagnosis confirmation by treatment response has its flaws. This is not to obviate the prompt administration of medications to relieve symptoms or treat illnesses. We would not quibble with using antibiotics to arrest infection, even if the lab test has not arrived or been conclusive. Seasonal sniffles and congestion may warrant a nasal spray even before or without rigorous allergy testing.

The current wave of positive responses to the new weight-loss drugs seems to have encouraged a "brain disease by success" mentality. The thinking goes like this: *I've struggled to lose weight for years and have been unsuccessful (and miserable) on a sustainable, consistent basis. On the new weight loss medication, I've lost weight, reduced my appetite, and think less compulsively about food. The medication affects my liver, pancreas, and gut hormones as well as their signals to my brain; therefore, I must have a brain disease that was lacking proper diagnosis and treatment.*

Can you recognize the flaws in this line of reasoning? Let's also add that the weight-loss drugs slow down digestive transit time, which leaves food in the stomach much longer. Of course, this feeling of fullness signals to the brain that eating more is no longer of interest. This is a very helpful outcome—but it is *normal* for the brain to respond this way, not evidence of a disease.

And What's More . . .

Hunger is not a disease! We are mammals, first and foremost. Yes, we've got a lot more going on than animals who hunt in the wild; but remember, mammals think about food constantly. It's wired into our survival.

Consider also that behavior itself, even destructive behavior, is not a disease (though its consequences may lead to disease). Eating behaviors are patterns largely conditioned by learned payoffs to the relief of internal crises provoked by neurophysiological dysregulation.

I resonate with those who admit: *I'm not even done with breakfast, but*

I'm thinking about what's for lunch. I get it—me too. Much of this is normal, but some of it is not.

Constant preoccupation with and dwelling upon food and eating originates with the longstanding habit of reward deficiency in digestive satiety. In common parlance, we can't get our mind off food because we lack the routine experience in our gut (starts there) and our brain that we are satisfied, we have had enough, we are not missing out, and we won't feel better if we eat more. Because of our evolutionary roots, overeating now is vestigial and maladaptive.

The basis of the "food noise" is the problematic and disruptive lack of blood sugar maintenance that afflicts the majority of people. Inadequate blood sugar regulation is *the* culprit in a multitude of health diseases and disorders, including and especially obesity. Due to evolutionary programming (it's in our genes to store calories just in case), diets of unnatural and highly processed foods, and the constant roller coaster of uneven blood sugar, the brain is provoked and commandeered into thinking about, planning, and seeking food. This is a normal combination of biochemical, cognitive, and behavioral responses to a lifetime of dysregulated and dissatisfied eating.

People overeat out of boredom (underarousal), emotional overload and stress (overarousal), and because the foods themselves are engineered and processed to cause cravings, overindulgence, and addiction. Sugar, salt, fat, taste additives, and the habit of addressing stress through food may trick us into eating until "food coma" shutoff kicks in. This is a maladaptive anxiety-reducing and sedating response. Unfortunately, it's often accompanied by self-criticism and self-derogation.

Notwithstanding these factors, the problem—and the solution—is the regulation and controlled maintenance of the digestive biome through hormone balance and blood sugar regulation. Along with such gastric regulation, the brain must become more regulated in its neuronal transmission to reduce high-alert vigilance in which anxiety is mediated by thinking about and seeking food as a reward.

This leads us into an exciting new world of good news: modern weight-loss drugs go a long way toward correcting the imbalances suffered by tens of millions.

In sum, rest assured that you are not diseased if or because you crave food, love food, and think about it constantly. These are normal responses to the dysregulated states of deprivation you have endured for so many years.

Extensive preoccupation with food (unless you are in the food industry) is annoying overkill and stretches the limits of normal mental balance. But it's not a brain disease. It's your gut signaling relentlessly to your brain that you are not satisfied and that something's not right. When there's a fire and the alarm is pulled, don't blame the fire department.

Remember also (in the words of my wise father), "Opinions come easily on a full stomach." Your brain and stomach should work harmoniously instead of vying in conflict for who is slave and who is master.

Obesity reflects an ongoing internal crisis of neurophysiology, a battle for self-regulatory control with hormonal normalcy and functionality.

When you look in the mirror, do you see a sick person? Someone with a bad, diseased brain? Or do you see a person who is sick and tired of being frustrated and stuck after years of earnestly putting forth effort to achieve goals with eating and weight?

You can stop blaming yourself, ascribing character flaws to your failed attempts, comparing yourself negatively and incessantly, and instead reject the idea that you have a diseased brain just because you like to eat and enjoy feeling satisfied. Your internal house is out of order. Let's clean it up and maintain the digestive and metabolic housekeeping.

I'll keep reminding you: You are a worthy person, a person of infinite value, someone who deserves to feel good about yourself and to see fruitful results from your intention and hard work.

My intention and effort in writing this book is to help you achieve goals along those lines—to have a more peaceable and healthy relationship with your mind, body, and with food, regardless of how many pounds you lose along the way.

And if you follow the simple (perhaps not always easy, but they are simple and straightforward) steps I outline, I promise you will lose weight.

Let's get started with practical information and plans to make you healthier, happier, and looking and feeling much better.

Next we look at the possibilities and promise of some new weight-loss medicines that can help you jumpstart your program.

CHAPTER 7

Blood Sugar and Metabolism

The Brain-Gut Connection

Are You Hungry?

One might think that eating is simply the natural response to hunger; but of course, it's more complicated than that! In addition to satisfying hunger, we may eat out of boredom, habit, in response to delicious aromas and presentation, or simply because food is available. We are barraged with food ads and enticements, we pass by restaurants and stores that beckon us to their tastes and aromas, social occasions include refreshments and meals, and of course we keep foods in our homes.

Though eating is a normal and necessary part of life, the feedback loop in our biology can often be less than healthy or functional. Many cues dangle temptations and invitations to eat. We can get into habits of overeating, eating when we're not truly hungry, and eating substances that are unhealthy and are not even "real" foods.

A key driver in our eating is how our blood sugar affects us. Understanding and gaining management and control of blood sugar is vital to maintaining or controlling weight, avoiding disease, feeling satisfied, and developing a more normal relationship with food, our appetite, and our body.

41

Brain, Gut, and Metabolism

Overeating, appetite and impulse problems, weight gain, and consequent metabolic effects are factors that "feed" into each other. Each amplifies the disorder of the others. Science has identified hormones and neurotransmitters that regulate appetite and satiety. Genetics, culture, habit, advertising, food availability, cost, taste, stress, time, and other factors play into what we eat, how much, and what it takes to satisfy physiological urges and mental desires.

Along with obesity, many Americans are beset with concerning proportions of metabolic disorders. Many of us suffer from high blood pressure, high cholesterol, fatigue and sleep problems, blood sugar and vascular problems, and a host of other health issues that chip away at well-being, longevity, and quality of life. Approximately three quarters of the adult population can be medically classified as metabolically abnormal. We are a sedentary, technologically indulged, and comfort-conditioned society. We are challenged to compensate and work with nature as well to forestall her encroachment as best and as long as we can.

Importance of Blood Sugar

As discussed in Chapter 2, hunger and health depend pivotally on the management of blood sugar. Our bodies are finely tuned to digest foods and convert them to energy. A precarious balance exists between releasing sugar into the bloodstream and counteracting it with insulin. Too little sugar in the system results in hypoglycemia and feeling weak and shaky. Too much sugar overloads the organs and causes a cyclical rebound effect of a temporary energetic sugar high, followed by a rebound or "crash" in which the body craves more sugar quickly. On this uncomfortable and unhealthy rollercoaster is where most Americans spend their days and appetites. Over time, too much blood sugar causes the body to become insulin resistant, a condition in which the insulin produced by the pancreas is insufficient to counteract and balance blood sugar. Eventually, this results in diabetes.

Processed foods, and especially simple carbohydrates (which the body converts to sugar), provide quicker fuel; but they burn quickly, leaving us hungry and craving. Complex carbs (such as those found in legumes, vegetables, and some fruits) break down more slowly, as do proteins. Three ounces of fish or chicken or beans is much more satisfying and energy producing than three ounces of chips or bread.

It's easy to become addicted to the tasty ingredients in processed foods, notably loaded with sugar, fat, and salt—the big three that hook us by evolutionary predisposition and by habit. These foods cause changes in the brain and the gut, thereby conditioning our appetites, blood sugar responses, and behaviors. Blood sugar problems cause disorder and eventually result in diseases.

Over the last two decades the medical criteria for blood sugar and blood pressure have become much more stringent, and more adults visiting physicians are apt to be labeled either diabetic or prediabetic. While this may be prudent for avoiding disease onset or progression, it does categorize a higher percentage of the population as metabolically disordered. The recommendations and prescriptions for drugs to control these conditions have drastically increased.

It's Personal

Diabetes runs in my family. Many relatives had it in addition to my mother who lost both legs due to progressive diabetes. As my own blood sugar began to climb (despite my dietary care), I became concerned and consulted my physician. He acknowledged that the statins I need to take (for cholesterol) may elevate blood sugar somewhat. However, he recommended a *semaglutide* to lower my systemic sugar.

After several months on this medication, I reduced my blood sugar, my lab blood work was better, and I lost even more weight faster than I was losing before. My exercise of "pushaways" (pushing away the plate of food) increased, and I found myself remarkably satisfied with a significantly smaller volume of food. I always remember my decades-long habit of ordering several entrees, just because I didn't want to miss anything. (This self-concept has gradually altered.)

Another benefit I experienced is that my taste and appetite for fattening food has decreased. I simply prefer lighter food with more protein and fiber. When I do eat pasta with sauce or fried foods, I tolerate much less before feeling like I don't want more. This change in my appetite and desires is a welcome enhancement. My physician was pleased with my positive response to semaglutide, but he also commended me on my dietary efforts. I remain very encouraged.

As a neuropsychologist, I understand, educate others, and practice the essentials of habit change, step by step with careful successive approximations.

Inch by inch, life's a cinch; yard by yard, life is hard. ~John Bytheway

Nothing succeeds like success itself—progress provides reinforcement and encouragement, along with renewed motivation. This notwithstanding, I was surprised at my seemingly effortless parallel change in food choices. I didn't expect these new habits to be so natural.

The Gut-Brain Connection

The gut is now known as the "second brain" in scientific circles. The gastrointestinal tract evolved with its own nervous system, the *enteric nervous system* (ENS). The "gut-brain axis" is a bidirectional neurohormonal communication system that is regulated through the central nervous system and the enteric nervous system[2]. This axis is fundamental to digestion, including gut microbes, propulsion along the colon, and feedback to the brain.

A proliferation of research studies and scientific articles document the delicate feedback relationship between our brain and digestive system. This already-known intimate connection will likely become increasingly foundational in the treatment of weight and associated medical conditions.

The natural interrelationship between brain and gut does not suggest disease of the brain as a basis of obesity. Nonetheless, scientific validity and prudence lead us to view hunger, weight, appetite, and metabolic problems as fundamentally physiological in origin with correlates in emotional

---

2. Hadhazy, Adam. "Think Twice: How the Gut's "Second Brain" Influences Mood and Well-Being." *Scientific American.* Feb 12, 2010. https://www.scientificamerican.com/article/gut-second-brain/

and behavioral tendencies. By intervening effectively to regulate and control the underlying physiology of gastrointestinal processes *and brain functions*, we can exert better leverage in succeeding with the management and mastery of neurophysiological, metabolic, mental/emotional, and behavioral control.

CHAPTER 8

The New Weight-Loss Medications

The Game Changers

The past century has welcomed many innovative inventions. This progress has accelerated in the recent decades. Some of these are game changers. Among the notable examples are: the internet, smart phones, birth control, vaccines that have helped to eradicate certain disease, airplanes and cars. I'm reminded of a 1988 TV commercial for General Motors, touting its new Cutlass model. The catch phrase was, "This is not your father's Oldsmobile."

We can add new weight-loss drugs to the list of game changers. These are not your mother's diet pills.

Previous medications for weight loss were mostly amphetamines. They had deleterious side effects, including damage to the heart. They proved ineffective for sustained weight loss and management. Amphetamine variations prescribed for weight loss have serious and harmful side effects. Though they suppress appetite, they are also highly addictive and destructive to organs, most notably the heart. And amphetamines are *very bad* for the brain.

Medications now being used to promote weight loss originated about twenty years ago and are still being prescribed for the treatment of diabetes, a progressive and devastating disease for many millions of Americans, and its incidence is sharply increasing. These newer medications have also shown to have synergistic positive side effects that are helpful for weight loss. The revolution in the pharmacology of blood sugar and appetite control has occurred and is evolving. Research continues to show that these newer meds also demonstrate protective effects for heart health. An accumulation of studies indicates that, for those with cardiovascular risk factors, these medications reduce the incidence and risk of cardiac events and strokes.[3]

How These Drugs Work

The new medications, which belong to a class called *glucagon agonists*, mimic the action of a hormone called glucagon-like peptide 1 (GLP-1). When blood sugar starts to rise after eating, these drugs stimulate the pancreas to produce more insulin. This extra insulin helps lower blood sugar (glucose) levels, which are important to prevent and control diabetes (Type 2). "GLP-1 also slows gastric emptying, suppresses appetite, improves satiety, decreases inappropriate glucagon secretion, and promotes beta-cell proliferation. GLP-1 receptor agonists have also demonstrated the ability to restore insulin secretory functions, thereby contributing to improvements in glycemic control and body weight reduction in diabetic patients."[4] The short-acting formulations work by delaying gastric emptying, thus reducing postprandial glucose levels. The long-acting agents affect both fasting and postprandial glucose levels.

Evidence suggests roles that GLP-1 analogs can play on receptors expressed throughout the human body, including reducing blood pressure, improvement in endothelial and myocardial function, recovery of failing and ischemic heart, arterial vasodilation, and increased diuresis and natriuresis.

---

3. Dagli, N., S. Kumar, R. Ahmad, M. Narwaria, and M. Hague. "An Update on Semaglutide Research: A Bibliometric Analysis and a Literature Review." PMC PubMed Central, Cureus 15(10) Oct 5 2023. https://www.ncbi.nlm.nih.gov/pmc/articles/PMC10552354/
4. Latif; W., Katerina J. Lambrinos; Preeti Patel, and Rolando Rodriguez. (2024). Compare and Contrast the Glucagon-Like Peptide-1 Receptor Agonists (GLP1RAs). NIH National Library of Medicine. https://www.ncbi.nlm.nih.gov/books/NBK572151/

The latest medications in this newer class used to treat insulin resistance and blood sugar excesses are various versions of *semaglutide* and *tirzepatide*. They are marketed under brand names like Ozempic, Wegovy, Mounjaro, Zepbound, and others. Semaglutide and tirzepatide are being studied closely for additional benefits to the heart, and new drugs are in development and emerging for medical use as well.

To understand the mechanism of action associated with these, we must look for a moment at how the body normally responds to food. When a healthy person eats food, the digestive tract sends a variety of chemical signals that engage elements of the endocrine and other systems to prepare the body to digest the food in the most efficient and beneficial manner possible. For best results, the blood sugar and lipid-related cholesterol compounds in the blood must maintain tight regulation through this process. Appropriate transport through the digestive system is also critical so that secretions of stomach acids and bile happen in the proper sequence, matching the stages of food breakdown timing with maintenance of beneficial bacteria at correct locations on the pathway. Further, the body systems must find a way to determine and regulate what type and how much food the digestive system can handle.

One key signaling chemical is glucagon-like peptide (GLP-1). When food is eaten, this compound acts to get the pancreas to boost insulin to prevent a blood sugar spike that would otherwise occur and simultaneously get the liver to reduce glucagon production. Glucagon acts to boost blood sugar as part of the sugar regulation system. GLP-1 also interacts with peristalsis, digestive transport, gastric emptying, as well as regulating lipid absorption, and further interacts with feelings of satiety, defining when enough nutrition has been acquired.

In the case of malfunctioning processes like diabetes and obesity, there may be an insufficiency in the GLP-1 signal pathway related to balancing the amount of food eaten versus the body's metabolic needs; overeating is a result of the imbalance. Pharmaceutical researchers, suspecting that the GLP-1 signal pathway might not be working effectively, looked for ways to enhance this signal. After much research, they found that a certain kind of iguana venom could act as a synthetic GLP-1 *agonist variant*, meaning it would bind to the same signal receptors that natural GLP-1 engage with and create an increased receptor response based on the dose given.

This discovery launched a large family of GLP-1 agonists. Semaglutide, and tirzepatide, these latest offerings in this family, effectively amplify all the GLP-1 signaling. The effect of the signal is to experience fullness sooner, positively reducing food intake. This caloric reduction effectively lowers long-term blood sugar, bringing about multiple metabolic, cardiovascular, and neuroprotective advantages.[5] Normal metabolic control is brought closer, and insulin requirements as well as resistance are both reduced.

Some of these drugs have another gastrointestinal hormone that complements GLP-1 by stimulating the activity of endocrine glands. GLP-2 promotes intestinal mucosal function. Some clinical trials have also shown GLP-2 may have therapeutic effects in the treatment of inflammatory bowel disease.

Unlike drugs used to modify state of mind (psychiatric drugs for depression, anxiety, sleep, attention, etc.) these newer blood sugar drugs target digestive absorption as well as the endocrine response in the liver and pancreas. They do not affect mental state (except insofar as modulating unbridled hunger that is seen in stress and addictive eating). Taking such a medicine to control metabolism is an assist (like an electric bike motor) to facilitate and enhance the main thrust of self-initiated forward progress.

An important caution when taking any of these medications for weight loss is the necessity to simultaneously be eating a healthy low-carb, high protein diet along with regular physical exercise to prevent muscle mass loss.

Unexpected Benefits

The synergistic actions of glucagon agonists are very effective in lowering and controlling blood sugar and suppressing appetite. Blood sugar modulation is critical for normal metabolic functioning, including countering the effects of insulin resistance, the main culprit in diabetes. Insulin resistance causes the bloodstream to become less responsive to insulin, the counterbalance to too much blood sugar.

---

5. Including potential protection from dementia.

Additionally, these medications slow down digestive transit time—the speed at which food moves through the digestive tract. Food remains in the stomach longer, causing a feeling of fullness and relaying to the brain that hunger is diminished. Thus hunger is no longer a priority, as satiety increases and lasts longer. Surprising and common to people on these meds is how they feel full on a fraction of the amount of food they are normally used to eating.

As more clinical evidence surfaces about these drugs, there appears to be a "dark horse" effect that is unexpected and amazing: people report marked reductions in cravings for alcohol and/or recreational drugs and pain medications. Neither researchers nor patients were prepared for this. The mechanism underlying this finding is not apparent; but this clearly needs further scrutiny and investigation.

If the glucagon agonists can simultaneously promote weight loss and treat addictions, they would indeed be even more revolutionary!

My Experience

My weight-loss journey has comprised several strategies, including the use of the new medications. In addition to losing pounds and normalizing my blood health, I have experienced some welcome side benefits regarding appetite and food.

I don't use drugs or alcohol, so those cravings are not an issue for me. However, everyone who struggles with weight and eating contends with cravings. I tend to prefer (and crave) savory foods over sweets. I love fried foods. Since taking such medicine, my yearning for and tolerance of fatty foods has dramatically reduced.

I have gotten used to eating much smaller amounts. Whereas I used to eat a bag or more of onion rings, I now am satisfied with one or two rings (if I eat them at all). I don't know that I will ever completely abandon my relationship with pizza; I used to eat four or six slices at a sitting, but now I eat one slice, maybe two, and I am done!

Also—and much to my further amazement—my desire for fatty and rich foods has markedly decreased. Not only do I not have a yen for them, but when I do eat fatty foods, I don't feel as good as when I eat less dense and more natural and nutritious substances. My body (the parts of me that are *teaching* my brain) show me through repetition and modification that vegetables and legumes *feel better* than heavy carbs and fats. Over time, I have even shifted my tastes to prefer less mayonnaise, sauces, and salad dressings. *Amazing!*

Another example of what I have come to believe over the years of my professional practice is that matter over mind is more powerful (and extant) than mind over matter. Will power lags far behind skill power and physiology in the quest for mastery and self-control.

We develop our self-image and self-concept through many inputs and experiences over time. I've heard it said that "inside a fat person is a thin person waiting to emerge." My thinner person has emerged, as has my ability to follow through and implement the healthful practices I have known about since adolescence.

However, appetites and perceived need die hard. I still order and buy more food than I can eat. I continue to modify old habits with increasing success. The days of ordering multiple entrees at restaurants are behind me. Now it's common for me to wrap up my leftovers at most meals or offer them to those around me (Sorry, Fido, not you).

Clearly, my brain, body, and habits are undergoing progressive transformation. I believe that my stomach looks at food and eating differently with whatever vision it uses. Because of my habit growing up of seeking and eating copious amounts of food, my father characterized me as having "big eyes" and a "hollow leg." (A metaphor for where the food goes in those who consume copiously.)

I put on lots of weight over the years, not because of a brain disease, but because of a disconnect in my neurophysiology. I was a sitting duck for undisciplined greed and excessive hedonism fostered and opportunized by the plentiful availability of unhealthy and addictive foods.

Training my brain through neuropsychological methods and giving my body a "pedal assist" to move my metabolism on the right direction has made huge differences in my health and my understanding about more complexities and wonders of the mind-body relationship.

I am very thankful for the medical breakthroughs that have benefited me with the blessings of the weight-loss drugs (and other medicines, as needed). The glucagon agonists act on my stomach rather than my brain. In that sense, my cerebral leader is more of a follower. But overall, my brain is happier to be a benchwarmer in this fortuitous journey. My brain still likes to think it's in charge (with many exceptions, like willpower); but it is pleased to follow what leads to satisfaction.

Remember: *opinions come easily on a full stomach*—as do many better choices.

Drawbacks

Medications typically have side effects. In deciding whether to use them, one must evaluate the costs and benefits. In some cases, significant negative side effects must be tolerated because the medicines are needed for a health issue of great crisis, threat, or priority. In many instances, we are allowed more discretion and take medications electively while determining their advantages and negative effects.

Weight-loss medications are elective. They do have side effects and are not appropriate for some people. They are contraindicated for patients who have a family history of certain cancers and for those with pancreas or kidney problems. It is important to see a licensed physician to determine if you are a candidate.

Some of the common side effects of these meds are gastrointestinal symptoms. These may include diarrhea, cramps, bloating, vomiting, constipation, or nausea. There have been rare reports of *gastroparesis*. This is a very unusual but serious condition in which the muscles of the stomach become intermittently paralyzed and generally weakened, leaving food in the stomach undigested. It is a rare but serious overreaction to the slowed transit time induced by the glucagon agonist medications. The reported rate of gastroparesis in semaglutide users is 0.01 percent.

In my own use, I experienced diarrhea and severe stomach cramps during the first few months I took these medications. I also had constipation. The occurrences were infrequent, very uncomfortable, and lasted several hours. I had approximately one bout per month for about five months. My body then got used to the meds, and these symptoms are no longer an issue.

These weight loss drugs are expensive. Without insurance coverage, they can cost $1,000 to $2,000 per month. Insurance companies are often reluctant to cover the cost. A physician can assist with a diagnosis that is approved for these prescriptions. Sometimes the doctor must jump through the hoops of *prior authorization* with the insurance carrier. Having a good relationship with a doctor who will help and advocate for you is needed.

Wegovy and Zepbound have been approved for weight loss. Ozempic and Mounjaro may be hard to get covered unless you have a diabetes diagnosis.

Another consideration is that you may need to continue these medications for years in order to control your weight. The jury is still out on whether weight loss can be sustained when going off the meds. Reports are that a significant percentage of users regain some weight when they stop the meds.

The popularity of these weight-loss drugs has spawned numerous telehealth sites where you can be interviewed online and receive a prescription. Due to the popularity of the drugs, there have been shortages while the makers ramp up production. To fill in the gap, compounding pharmacies have made and sold their own versions of semaglutide and tirzepatide. I caution you to be wary of these imitations, as the makers often add their own ingredients; thus purity cannot be assured. The internet provides opportunities to obtain "look-alikes" cheaply, even without a prescription. I caution against this as well. See a licensed physician. Do it right and protect yourself.

As of this writing, two pharmaceutical companies produce these drugs: Novo Nordisk makes Ozempic and Wegovy: Eli Lilly makes Mounjaro and Zepbound. I predict a proliferation of these and newer weight-loss drugs implementing this biochemical methodology in the coming years. The medications will be better and cheaper, easier to get, and eventually covered by insurance regularly. The handwriting is on the wall. These newer medications are a godsend for helping many people lose weight. But they cannot by themselves alter lifestyle and develop healthier habits. The rest is up to each of us.

Weight-Loss Medications Need Teammates and Coaches

As I have elucidated previously in this book and in my other writings and opinions, it is incomplete and ineffective to address many organic somatic conditions through medication alone or counseling support. It is necessary to treat the organs in deficiency or dysregulation (brain, stomach) while also providing collateral support as needed, or as helpful.

Weight-loss drugs may be wonderful, and you may lose weight (up to a point) somewhat effortlessly. But you must also change your diet, your habits, your relationship with your body and with food. You must become better at dealing with stress and negative emotions. You must learn about healthy eating in order to gradually modify your diet without incurring the deprivation that will likely make you revert. You must learn to accept and love yourself more based on who you are and what you do, rather than on what you look like or what other people think or say.

Remember: you are incredibly precious and special, regardless of what you weigh, what you eat, or how you look.

Toward these ends, I have developed a comprehensive weight-loss program that works, whether or not you use the "pedal assist" of weight-loss drugs.

CHAPTER 9

Food Addictions

A ddictions have been associated stereotypically with drugs and alcohol, but the understanding of addictions has widened in recent years to incorporate food. To include food in the addictions category may seem odd because, unlike drugs or alcohol, food is required for survival. So what's this about foods being addictive?

Though food is necessary, and healthy foods are nourishing, even foods that are "good" can have adverse effects, depending upon how our bodies react to them and how much of particular foods we eat. An evidentiary dynamic is at work. By habitually eating foods that affect us adversely, we can paradoxically develop strong cravings for foods that push our bodies from helpful nutritional absorption into maladaptive reactions. Propensities for food addictions are multiplied with unhealthy, ultra-processed foods that comprise the diets of so many Americans.

To put this into context, let's review the basics of addictions and review examples and explore parallels to the problems with addictions.

The Nature of Addiction

The term "addiction" is often used rather loosely, which sometimes leads to misunderstanding. For example, some postulate addiction to sports or books. But this questionable terminology is meant to indicate a strong or intense fondness for sports or books. However, in a psychological and medical sense, the term "addicted" has the clear implication of indicating a problem that *interferes* to some degree with a person's life, functioning, health, or well-being. To call natural, wholesome, and healthy feelings an addiction is not reasonable. To feel good physically and mentally naturally, without drugs, is a sign and a consequence of good general health.

For a significant percentage of the US population, addiction is front and center in its stranglehold upon health and productive functioning. Whether an addiction involves a substance or a destructive behavior, many in its throes are somewhere in the cycle of thinking about either indulging, actually indulging, or recovering from indulgence.

Addictions are complex syndromes that afflict health, include the development of maladaptive behaviors and dependencies, and typically impair functioning in relationships, productivity, and self-care for millions. Addictions weaken self-confidence and self-esteem, bring conflicts and negative emotions, and erode our sense of responsibility for the resulting dysfunction that follows. Central to any addiction are problems with self-management, self-control, obsessive thinking, and neurological dysregulation.

Addiction also goes hand in hand with anxiety. The brain and nervous system in states of disrepair and deprivation due to addiction is anxious, biologically as well as psychologically. Since most people live under conditions of great stress and duress (internal and environmental), and the development of adequate coping resources and self-regulation mechanisms is challenging, many rely upon substances or behaviors that blunt the pain and negative emotions and provide temporary escape. This inevitably creates maladaptive habits that reinforce the problem and further erode our coping skills.

Addictions develop and involve compulsive indulgence in substances such as drugs, foods, and behaviors (including eating behaviors). Current trends and supporting research highlight an emerging awareness of food addiction as more people develop health problems that are directly related to what they eat. Biological, economic, and sociological influences collude to encourage us to eat too much and consume foods that eventually make us sick.

The food-processing industry has come under scrutiny for advanced manufacturing and marketing that manipulate our inherent attraction (and resulting addiction) to fat, sugar, and salt. The wide availability of unnatural and cheap foods pander to immediate gratification and take advantage of genetic programming that predisposes us to unwitting caloric storage. A multitude of social, political, and economic influences keep millions of people unable to provide adequately for themselves and families, which creates a sure recipe for many kinds of addictions. Addictions are pervasive, adhering to determinants that are biological, social, destructive, and essentially contagious, i.e., via peers and life pressures, not unlike microbes.[6]

The propensity to become addicted is practically wired into our need to escape pain, reduce stress, and quell anxiety. This does not mean that addiction is inevitable. But addiction is a likely cohort of anxiety that is facilitated by poor resilience, vulnerable lifestyles, and a lack of adequate resources and interventions to protect ourselves, weather adversity and conflict, and develop adequate sustainable self-regulation, self-soothing mechanisms, and overall self-control.

Before focusing on food addictions, it's helpful to understand how addictions work, how they intertwine with emotional and biochemical processes, and how they compare with habits.

The Addiction-Anxiety Connection

Addiction is a dependency on some substance or activity that causes some degree of harm to, or interference with, a person's life. The dependency is powered by the tranquilizing (i.e., anxiety masking) effect of the substance or activity.

All addictions originate from anxiety and are responses to relieving (or masking) anxiety. The seminal role of anxiety in forming and sustaining addictions doesn't negate or omit the biology of physiological dependence on certain substances, or the build-up of tolerance. Clearly, the brain becomes

---

6. While obviously involving microbes, diseases such as AIDS and hepatitis are among those spread by addictions.

accustomed to some chemicals (such as opiates or alcohol) in a manner that creates physiological withdrawal and the possibility of severe illness or death if withdrawal is too acute or sudden. The pernicious and stubborn recurrence of anxiety develops a cycle of addiction and withdrawal in the first place that can easily lead to physiological dependence in addition to more pervasive anxiety.

Addiction generates the belief that the addicted person cannot live without the necessary substance/object/behavior. In such cases, the challenge to conquering addictions involves instituting a safe and viable way of *eliminating anxiety*. Once this is in place, habits can be changed, along with revising the belief that one *must* engage or indulge in the desires that propel the addictive substance or behavior.

Anxiety is a painful emotion to experience and is worsened when it has no apparent cause and resurfaces repeatedly without "logical' provocation. Anxious people feel bad due to the anxiety, and feel worse when the emotion seems to make no sense.

If an anxious person can "take" something or do something that blocks awareness of the anxiety, they feel tremendous relief. The relieved person feels calm, serene, tranquilized, and temporarily free of the agonizing feeling of anxiety. The relief feels so good that it makes a profound impression on the body and mind. Though many addicts are aware of the sequence of actions leading to addiction, not every addict is aware of the process *while* it is occurring. This sequence happens to each addict at a profound level of being, regardless of the conscious awareness.

The process of addiction creates a state of self-sabotage in the addict. This makes it especially difficult to overcome the addiction because the addict is driven to engage in self-defeating activities, becoming one's own worst enemy.

We don't fully know why certain substances or activities mask anxiety. Some drugs appear to physically block our awareness of anxiety, via nervous system or brain neurotransmitters. Certain activities such as thumb-sucking or hair-pulling appear to be intrinsically soothing to some individuals, with the apparent comfort of the activity blocking awareness of their anxiety.

Habit and Addiction

Many people confuse habits and addictions despite the significant difference between the two. A *habit* is a behavior pattern that is so established in our behavioral repertoire that it is usually carried out regularly without conscious effort. Since a certain amount of effort goes into establishing a habit, a certain effort is typically required to change a habit.

A good example of a habit is how we train ourselves to automatically remove the car keys when we leave our car. When we go to a car wash, a car repair, or leave our car with a valet parking service, a special conscious effort is required in order to not walk off with the car keys.

When we make the conscious effort, many habits are not that difficult to change; the essence is remembering to be conscious about it. People sometimes mistake habits for addictions. The two can be coupled but have fundamental differences. With addiction, no matter how conscious one is, the addictive urge is rather compelling or overwhelming, depending upon the severity of the addiction.

Unlike most habits, addictions are extremely difficult to give up. The person is driven and compulsive. But in the case of habits, the person's actions represent highly learned activities that are often amenable to conscious efforts to change.

How Even "Healthy" Foods Can Become Addictive

Our bodies and minds get used to things. Whether it's novel experiences, environmental stimuli, or things we take into our body, our systems gradually adapt. This can be helpful or disadvantageous. A personal example serves to illustrate:

In 1980, I relocated from New York State to Los Angeles. I moved to Pasadena, a lovely city at the foothills of the San Gabriel Mountains. I was excited and delighted to be done with the snow and cold of the Northeast. Also, I had suffered severely for years from pollen allergies, especially ragweed that grows copiously in the summer months and causes hay fever. This plant doesn't grow in western states. *Ah,* no more hay fever—I could breathe in California! Los Angeles, however, is known for smog. This is especially bad in the city's surrounding inland valleys. Pasadena is among the areas notorious for smog, so thick that the mountains a half-mile away are not visible on some days.

When I first moved there, I could breathe. My hay fever cleared up and I didn't mind the smog. In fact, I ran miles every day without difficulty. However, gradually over time (about a year) I developed allergies to new pollens that grow in that area, and I again suffered significant allergic symptoms. The smog began to affect me, and on some days it choked my breathing.

Our bodies adapt—sometimes building immune responses with inflammation and at other times building a tolerance to what's absorbed. As I aged, it became necessary to take medications to control my blood pressure and cholesterol. My cardiologist told me that my body would get used to them, and he was right.

Now back to foods: We tend to repeatedly eat the foods that taste good and make us feel good. And these are often unhealthy foods. But even with healthy, nutritious foods, our body and brain become acclimated and eventually *expect* (desire, crave) to be satisfied and rewarded with foods to which we've become accustomed. We develop a type of withdrawal when these foods are withheld. This happens with "good" foods as well as junk foods. So where does the addiction enter?

Remember that addiction is a dependency on some substance or activity that causes a degree of harm to, or interference with, a person's life. The dependency is powered by the tranquilizing (i.e., anxiety masking) effect of the substance or activity. The problem with addiction to "healthy" foods arises when habitually eaten foods become toxic (in the energy sense) to the body and mind. This is surprisingly common even with nutritious foods like eggs, grains, and dairy, among others. A build-up in the gut and nervous system causes difficulties with neuronal regulation and smooth metabolism. This often results in psychological symptoms such as anxiety, depression, fears, and other symptoms. It can also cause or exacerbate brain fog and sleep problems.

I have treated many hundreds of patients with intransigent symptoms that are made worse by the foods they eat habitually. Though medical science is becoming more conversant with the effects of diet, these sensitivities are still well beneath their radar. People who test normally on food allergy tests can often have significant sensitivities to foods. We detect these sensitivities using Voice Technology. Then the solution involves identifying and avoiding or eliminating these foods from the diet. Improvements occur rapidly when following this regimen.

No one wants to be informed that some of their favorite ("good") foods are causing them problems. But this reality has been empirically established again and again.

So the bad news here is that you can become addicted to certain "healthy" foods if you eat too much of them or have a systemic sensitivity. The good news is that it's fixable, partly by the treatments discussed herein and partly by abstention from the offending substances (which may also include spices and flavorings).

Now for the "bad" foods . . .

A plethora of information and evidence shows that the proliferation and abundance of processed foods in our diets is killing us. Rather than talk about the food manufacturing industry per se, I focus here on the practical aspects of how processed food causes food addiction and compounds weight and health problems.

Insidious Bad Food Addictions

The energy-toxic reaction of typically healthy and nutritious foods causing unpleasant effects is a difficult concept to understand despite its demonstrable validity. Aside from food-specific reactions that some individuals have, a more prevalent problem is that the body and brain often begin to crave foods that we eat in excess. This is how the overload toxic effect develops and where the addiction arises. The more of these foods eaten, the more the gut and brain desire them. That can occur with any food.

The biochemistry of food addictions becomes more dire when unhealthy processed foods are eaten habitually. As the food industry refines its scientific methods of processing foods to maximize taste with addictive rewards from artificial, flavor-enhanced, and ultra-processed ingredients, the result is compounded. Chemicals that augment and maximize taste are blended with copious amounts of fat, sugar, and salt, along with artificial flavors and cheap additives shown to contribute to obesity, cancer, and other diseases and metabolic malfunctions. Artificial sweeteners and colors, flavor enhancers, preservatives, hydrogenated fats, and other ingredients are among the staple and cheaply produced foods that heighten taste stimulation and longer shelf life, and have the effect of hooking us—gut and brain—to crave more.

The food-processing industry has come under scrutiny for advanced manufacturing and marketing that manipulate to their advantage our inherent attraction (and resulting addiction) to fats, sweets, and salt. The wide availability of unnatural and cheap foods pander to immediate gratification and take advantage of genetic programming that predisposes us to unwitting caloric storage.

Eventually, as more of these "non-foods" are eaten, normal taste for real and nutritious food morphs into addictive cravings for fast, accessible, high-density and high-caloric substitutes for natural and nutritious real food. The result is an overload of calories, poor nutrition, obesity, metabolic and organ damage, and a vicious cycle of blood sugar rollercoaster that mires its victims in constant need to fulfill appetites that seek quick and frequent replenishment with very little lasting satisfaction.

Use This Information

Being armed with information about how our bodies and minds work and how they can be tricked or seduced by various foods can empower us to notice and control our physiology and habits more effectively. We are not victims or "bad" to be tricked in this way; we can use this knowledge to make better choices.

PART III

The Weight Control Program

CHAPTER 10

Control Your Mind and Body

W e all value and strive for the self-control that is natural and bi-ologically necessary. Along with accommodating fluctuations in our internal functions and balances, we gravitate toward a stable equilibrium or *homeostasis*, "the self-regulating process by which biological systems maintain stability while adjusting to changing external conditions."[7]

Some physiological functions require narrow tolerances to maintain health (such as body temperature), while others can fluctuate widely for long periods of time—but not without eventual deleterious health consequences. Some deviations can be subjectively undetectable as they progress to cause damage (e.g., blood pressure, cholesterol, atherosclerosis). Medical tests are needed to identify these "silent killers."

A multitude of effects and symptoms notify us when something doesn't feel right. We may eat something that causes gastric distress (such as bloating, diarrhea, etc.) or other symptoms, perhaps allergic reactions or mood changes. The complex and sensitive relationships we have with

---

7. Billman, George E. Homeostasis: "The Underappreciated and Far Too Often Ignored Central Organizing Principle of Physiology." *Frontiers in Physiology*: 2020; 11, 200.

food, our body, and eating patterns often become entwined with negative feelings we have about ourselves and our relationship to these issues.

Cravings, impulse control lapses, weight gain, mental focus, and organization are among the areas in which so many deviate from self-control and become major concerns in the domains of physical and mental health. They handily affect our self-image, relationships, spending habits, sleep, and other aspects of daily functioning.

How we eat—what, how much, when—is a critical part of self-control. We tend to think (and social forces reinforce this erroneous notion) that if we don't control our appetite and eating habits, we are failing in our will power and self-control. However, despite the need for personal responsibility, intention, commitment, and conscious management, other influences and propelling forces sway our choices.

Propelling Forces
Stress, anxiety, and preponderant negative emotions
With all the demands, responsibilities, environmental stressors, and our own individual proclivities in emotional and biological orientation and coping mechanisms, even the most regulated and disciplined people can sometimes become overwhelmed and vulnerable. Many lack adequate self-regulation and effective dietary and self-care habits.

When stress, anxiety, and other negative emotions pressure us to find relief, what type of relief is more convenient (and often justified) than eating? We all need to eat. Though food may serve as an escape, its general necessity and social validation can conceal its secondary value as a palliative for overwhelming feelings.

A physiological reality underlies the self-medicating effect of eating. "Comfort" foods (sugar, carbohydrates, and calorie-dense foods) flood the bloodstream quickly and supply the brain with "feel good" neurotransmitters. Food can serve as a safe release valve, absorbed in the routine of what we ordinarily do. But the habit of poor eating tends to creep up surreptitiously and gradually.

Blood sugar fluctuations and dips

Intricate and delicate biological mechanisms signal and regulate our brain, endocrine system, and organs to supply and control the flow of nutrients to our cells. These mechanisms release and store energy, promote cell growth and health, and excrete waste and toxins. A fundamental part of this process is the management of blood sugar.

Because food is there

When asked why he robbed banks, notorious criminal Willie Sutton said, "Because that's where the money is." Similarly, all too often, we eat simply because food is *there*. This parsimonious explanation underlies a lot of unnecessary consumption.

Our body responds to cues from our surroundings as well as internal metabolic affairs. When food is nearby and perhaps accompanied by the aromas, presentation, or sight of people eating, our senses are aroused; we may be cued to eat by signals that transcend or replace the actual hunger feeling.

Opportunities to eat are plentiful for most in the US. Though many people have trouble affording increasing prices, cheap food (usually processed food with dense calories) is available at low cost. The rituals of serving food and eating together typically accompany social events and get-togethers where food is everywhere. Temptation precedes and follows its appeal.

Boredom, habit, and fatigue

Mindless eating is a common pastime while watching TV or during social activities. We may graze on empty calories (such as snacks and processed foods) without limit, not noticing how much is consumed. We often eat just because "it's time to eat." We overeat out of habit or to fill the void from a lack of other satisfactions. Such eating beyond reasonable necessity can train our internal system to ignore when we are full.

Lack of sleep is correlated with overeating and weight gain. Rushing around through activities, inadequate hydration, no rest periods, and insufficient food intake throughout the day to steady blood sugar levels an easily result in overdoing the intake once you are home. Some people capitulate to "hangry" (angry and hungry) bouts and use food in abundance to calm down and self-soothe, sometimes even to mollify aggression. The self-regulation cues that signal *enough* can be dulled by fatigue.

Lack of exercise, irregular exercise, or too much exercise can lull or jolt the body and brain into misleading connection with true nutritional and volume needs. Being sedentary facilitates obtaining stimulation through the tongue and stomach.

Culture and tradition

Food is a paramount tradition with rituals and imperatives in many cultures and celebrations. Food accompanies family gatherings where eating a lot is expected. My father counseled me on how to "never let buffet restaurants make a profit on our family!" In human evolution, eating voluminously was needed whenever food was scarcer. Eating can be a way to express appreciation or respect or even convey material fortune.

Medications, drugs, and alcohol

Some medications are known to produce metabolic changes that include increased appetite and weight gain even as they may relieve disturbing and sometimes dangerous symptoms. Among these in particular are drugs for depression, anxiety, and psychosis. Such drugs exert powerful effects on neurotransmitters and hormones. Marijuana is known for inducing "the munchies." Alcohol tends to dull the senses (a significant attraction for some), but this includes a blunted sensitivity to and awareness of food intake.

The cause-and-effect trade-offs from overeating must be "weighed" against the benefits many foods and chemical substances offer. On balance, the warping of appetite and metabolic regulation are excellent reasons to develop a lifestyle of caring for our mental and physical health without reliance upon psychopharmacology or recreational intoxicants to manage ourselves and feel good.

Appeal the verdict, appease the appetite

The influences and combinations of emotional eating, food addictions, the blood sugar rollercoaster, and faulty self-care habits don't take long to fasten us to overeating patterns, weight gain, and reduced health. But it doesn't have to be this way!

We can counter these influences, engage more successfully with nature, and achieve better results. Notwithstanding the numerous genetic, environmental, and lifestyle factors that can undermine eating habits and weight control, changes almost anyone can make will improve health, self-control, and confidence. A core underpinning to defeat overeating is what I refer to as *gastro modulation*: the self-regulation of appetite, satiety, and metabolic balance. The practical multimodal program I designed, which allowed me to drop 105 pounds without deprivation or suffering, came from following these discoveries and applying them to a workable pattern.

Gastro modulation

Controlling blood sugar correlates with the self-regulation of appetite, satiety, and metabolic balance. While there is no substitute for healthy eating, emotional regulation, and self-control, their development may be assisted by some medications gaining attention as described in Chapter 8. A medically supervised regimen to manage blood sugar and reduce appetite can also be helpful for those who are good candidates. However, we are still faced with the challenge of managing our emotions, habits, attitudes, and diets. Toward this end, I offer the following solutions.

The Weight Control Program Components

This solid weight control program emphasizes a sensible life and brain balance, becoming friends with your brain and body, and developing a healthier and less compulsive relationship with food and eating. A summary of the program components:

1. **Neuronal regulation through EEG neurofeedback.**
   Training your brain with EEG neurofeedback will improve your overall brain health and make you mentally stronger, more durable, more flexible, and more resilient. Proven effective for a vast majority of people, neurofeedback reduces stress and improves sleep—two major factors in controlling appetite and weight. Along with relieving anxiety, depression, trauma, and other negative emotions, neurofeedback increases calmness and patience and modulates appetite and satiety by making your brain more aware

71

of your body. Eating yourself into self-loathing or "food stupor" is less likely when your brain is in tune with your body awareness.

2. **Voice Technology and Thought Field Therapy for cravings, negative emotions, and self-sabotage.**
   Voice Technology eliminates negative emotions, stress, intrusive thinking, shame, fear of failure, and other problems in minutes. The technique is also instrumental in correcting self-sabotage that interferes with motivation and successful behavior change. Since this can be done by phone, patients can have access to assistance more conveniently. And the self-help version of this treatment, called Thought Field Therapy, is an effective method as well.

3. **Behavior modification to control and change habits.**
   To observe, evaluate, and adjust responses through structured alterations in line with principles and schedules of reinforcement and extinction is far more effective for emotional or behavioral change. In this way I help patients use reliable methods of probability, frequency, intensity, and duration to end addictions and reduce unwanted behaviors while building adaptive ones.[8]

4. **Practical dietary wisdom, tips, and techniques.**
   My personal journey led me to discover and include many tips, tricks, and hacks to stabilize blood sugar and appetite and work around the temptations and traps that derail functional eating.

Examples:

- ✓ Drink lots of water.
- ✓ Pay attention to preparation, convenience, and proximity of meals.
- ✓ Add more food bulk with fewer calories.

---

8. Also outlined in my book, *Life Control: Take Charge and Get Ahead.*

✓ Reduce salt and enhance taste with spices and fresh, natural foods.
✓ Tame the salt/sugar/fat dragon by avoiding processed foods.
✓ Properly utilize temptation timeouts and probability methods.
✓ Control blood sugar by modulating fast-burn and slow-burn metabolism.

5. **Increased movement and smart exercise.**
Physical movement is crucial to facilitate faster metabolism, reduce stress, improve circulation, sleep better, and achieve improved well-being. Realistically, many people have mobility limits, physical impairments, or injuries that limit exercise. Though quite important, exercise plays less of a role in weight reduction than proper eating and metabolism balance.

Moving just a bit more on a regular basis (within one's physical limits) helps tremendously. Increase movement and/or exercise by 10 percent every two weeks. If you can walk ten blocks, stretch it to eleven. Aim for that *JND: just noticeable difference* in effort and tolerance. You'll be surprised to feel how your tolerance, mobility, and fitness improve, little by little.

6. **Focus on important relationships.**
As you strive to befriend your mind and body, include and integrate social relationships. We all need to practice tolerance, acceptance, and forgiveness of others and ourselves. Those around us share similar challenges and struggles. They may not say so, just as we may withhold our own embarrassments, anxiety, and inhibitions over self-control and body image. If you make yourself proximal, communicative, and emotionally available, you will notice increasingly that others value and accept you, just as they want validation, reassurance, and acceptance. Showing our availability, vulnerability, and imperfections will reveal how much more okay we are than what we may suspect. This also gives others implicit permission to

share their struggles with us. Everyone is up against nature, internally and externally. Why not share the struggle?

7. **Incremental diet changes and better choices day by day.**
Aim for incremental diet changes and better choices day by day. Bear in mind that lasting behavior change requires time and gradual adjustment. This is true for our body, our habits, and our self-concept. It's understandable to be eager to attain quick results; this is important for confidence and motivation.

I encourage you to look at the bigger picture with hope and positive expectations, and to embark on a self-control and reinvention journey with planning and patience. After all, you plan on living a long time, right?

If you try even a few of my recommendations, I promise that you will feel better physically and emotionally, and you will become more in control of your eating and relationship with food.

A poem for inspiration:

Hunger Is My Friend

Hunger is my friend
Who visits every day.
I welcome him and satisfy,
Then send him on his way.

Hunger can be stubborn
And can nag me like a child.
I need to teach him discipline
So he doesn't run too wild.

I meet with hunger joyfully
When we both follow rules.
I won't let his insistence
Deter me from my goals.

Hunger bows to cravings
To obtain what he wants now.
Withdrawal threatens savings
From my goals and best know-how.

My relationship with hunger
Must evolve from master/slave
Toward functional and orderly
To enjoy what I will have.

A Parallel

A pithy saying by Bill Clinton during his presidency, referring to his bottom-line summary of what was important and motivating to people concerning monetary relevance, was, "It's the economy, stupid!" To apply his summary wisdom in regard to our food consumption and weight (without the insult), *It's the gastronomy, friend!*

It's the food that makes us fat: plain and true, but far from simple.

The essential truth: eating problems and weight control are matters of brain, gut, genetics, and habit..

We need to fix the entire interconnected system, as best we can with as little belittlement, shame, self-degradation, suffering, and deprivation as possible.

The path I share is a solid plan that will work for most people, temporary setbacks and willpower struggles notwithstanding.

Now we can talk about the mechanics of how this all works.

CHAPTER 11

Self-Regulation— Physiological and Emotional

Our Internal Engine and Control Mechanisms

Human bodies utilize innate processes and feedback loop mechanisms to signal and control our blood sugar, appetite, satiety, and food desires. These mechanisms are dependent upon and reflective of gut biochemistry and its interaction with brain chemistry and awareness. Though overeating, obesity, and food obsessions are not attributable to brain disease, the case for *disorder* in the brain is strong. Various metabolic disorders that disrupt normal and adequate eating and weight maintenance, as well as a host of other disorders, are governed by the brain as a control center.

Although eating particular foods results in obesity, our neurological and emotional regulation and our ability to manage stress and deal with cravings and self-sabotage all affect our ability to make consistent choices and sustain habits that result in desired weight loss and maintenance. Knowledge of nutrition, food selection, reasonable exercise and movement, and healthy lifestyle habits are necessary—but *not sufficient*. Management of stress and neurophysiological and emotional regulation without suffering or deprivation are key to sustainable weight control.

Two powerful noninvasive techniques that I have used for many years help patients alleviate many of the symptoms and conditions that cause the greatest distress and dysfunction—EEG neurofeedback and Thought Field Therapy—are instrumental in promoting self-regulation and eliminating the traumatic underpinnings that throw people out of balance and influence poor eating and weight gain. The principles and applications of these interventions help a variety of disorders (including eating and weight issues). They reduce dysfunction, eliminate negative emotions, and build sustainable patterns of self-control.

Self-Regulation: The Inside Story of Brain Function

The powerful structure that sits atop our shoulders is a marvelous control center, governing how we feel and operate. Along with its sensitivity, our brain is capable of adjustments. Our brain's plasticity allows it to grow, change, modify, and improve its functioning. Self-regulation is how our brain manages our internal neurological affairs by channeling and integrating the firing of brain neurons—think of it as our interior EEG (electroencephalogram). This ordinary biological function is complex, elegant, intricate, and subject to many influences that can disrupt or *dysregulate* neurological function and cause many types of physiological and psychological problems. Developing and maintaining stable self-regulation is vital to reducing anxiety and keeping it at bay.

The body and brain's innate mechanisms that run our internal "housekeeping" include the maintenance of appropriate and modulated fight-or-flight responses, self-soothing mechanisms, alertness and relaxation, inhibition of overreaction and overarousal, and smooth transitions between "states" of arousal, waking, and sleeping. Disruptions in or faulty development of good self-regulation result in the body's mismanagement of metabolic functioning and/or subjective symptoms of discomfort. These can range from anxiety and depression to intense stress, sleep problems, headaches and other pain, digestive problems, weight gain, and a host of other health ailments that alert us when something is not right with our neuronal transmission and regulation.

Neuronal Regulation Through EEG Neurofeedback

Neurofeedback brain training is a particularly elegant and enduring method for the establishment and honing of the essential self-regulation and diminishing of symptoms such as anxiety. Training your brain with EEG neurofeedback improves overall brain health and makes you mentally stronger, more durable, flexible, and resilient.

Proven effective for a vast majority of patients, neurofeedback relieves negative emotions (i.e., anxiety, depression, and trauma) and reduces stress and improves sleep—major factors in controlling appetite and weight. We know that mindless eating goes hand in hand with dissociation between emotions and physiological satiety.

Neurofeedback increases calmness and patience and modulates appetite and satiety by making the brain more aware of the body. Eating yourself into a "food stupor" and self-loathing is far less likely when your brain is in tune with your body awareness.

To maximize its effectiveness, the brain needs valid real-time information to balance, stabilize, and regulate. Just as we see visually by looking outward (needing a mirror to see what's on our back), we process neurologically without direct access to the network of neurons firing inside our brain. Thus we need a mirror of sorts to witness how our brain fires in real time. Neurofeedback, or EEG biofeedback, is an effective (noninvasive and nonchemical) method for delving inside our brain to observe, monitor, and modify (if necessary) the firing of neurons and the flow of important information that affects our self-regulation.

This scientifically proven technique has been practiced clinically for more than a half-century to diminish anxiety and other psychological and physiological symptoms. This method of "training" our brainwaves actually improves our brain function and self-regulation and promotes better emotional and cognitive functioning. This technique induces beneficial and enduring results even when practiced for a short time.

What Is EEG Neurofeedback?

Neurofeedback is a form of self-regulation training, a natural process that is a necessary part of good brain function that permits the brain and central nervous system to function more capably, efficiently, and proficiently.

By taking advantage of the brain's ability to adapt (plasticity), EEG neurofeedback directly trains our brainwaves with the use of computers and specific, carefully calibrated software.[9] Working with a trained professional is recommended when beginning neurofeedback as this is a gradual learning process. Some people may eventually decide to perform their own training by obtaining their own equipment and applying the learning on themselves—similar to practicing at a gym with a trainer and then acquiring home equipment.

During neurofeedback training, electrical brain activity is measured by the electroencephalogram, and the patient (with practitioner guidance) observes the brain in action from moment to moment on a computer screen. With a benign adhesive, electrode sensors are attached to the scalp. Nothing goes into the head via these wires. The EEG sensors simply monitor and conduct the signal as a livestream from the head and brain to an amplifier and is displayed on one or more computer screens.

Brain signals are digitally transformed into audiovisual information, presented in the form of entertaining and engaging imagery. Watching a movie or game is used to attract interest and keep the patient focused on the screen. The marvel of electronics makes it possible to watch or "play" a game (usually for about thirty minutes at a time) by actually controlling it with our brainwaves. The efficacy of this process lies in the filtering of our brainwaves and in the science of selecting the range of signals that our brain needs to alter in order to feel and function better. The feedback we receive occurs as the game goes better, seemingly on its own.

Digital special effects show live feedback information that illustrates how much and how often the brain is "in the zone" according to individually set filters and parameters determined together by the patient and the therapist. The feedback, which encompasses thousands of subtle signals per session, gently encourages and rewards the brain for spending more brainwave time within the specified ranges.

This effortless brain exercise is the critical agency of the effects. The brain is subtly coached to make more of certain brainwaves and fewer of

---

9. EEG biofeedback is the training of brainwaves. Another more localized and limited type of biofeedback, called EMG biofeedback (electromyogram) is used to train specific muscles.

others, which is, in part, a form of *operant conditioning*—a behavioral term for the strategic use of reinforcement that conditions the brain and nervous system in a safe, subtle, and persistent way with the result that those behaviors become more probable.

Because the operant conditioning model does not account for the vast transforming changes that routinely occur with a newer *infra-low frequency (ILF) neurofeedback* training modality called *endogenous neuromodulation*, we have advanced our understanding of how the brain integrates its own information as it observes it in real time. This model is characterized by the absence of reinforcers but still relies on a complementary inhibiter design that marks different levels and steps in the process that identify the state of the brain's dysregulation.

Any response to this information, including any prescription for change, is left to the discretion of the brain. Consider this guiding principle from neuroscientist Paul Bach-y-Rita: "If you give the brain any information about itself, it will make sense out of it."

As the brain monitors, adjusts, and improves self-regulation, greater internal functioning and modulation occurs, and the brain transitions to *practice* more of its newfound regulation balance and homeostasis. This results in new perceptions, new adaptive habits, improved attitudes and expectations, and augmented flexibility. Better self-regulation becomes the brain's "new normal." This new functioning is reinforced through the repetition of more adaptive habits and the inherent and external rewards experienced as a result of improved brain and behavioral functioning.

The fundamental distinction between operant conditioning and endogenous neuromodulation is that the former only engages with macroscopic phenomena—operant conditioning only works well when the rewarded events stick out above the normal variability of the signal. Good regulation is a matter of greater subtlety that is only available in feedback via endogenous neuromodulation.

Using an exercise model relevant to neurofeedback as "taking your brain to the gym neurologically," we become more fit by subjecting the body to the gradual structured challenges of physical exercise. Our body adapts and gradually becomes stronger, more durable, flexible, and resilient, and with easier recovery.

When we challenge our heart, lungs, and muscles, we are simply inducing and strengthening physiological responses. The practice and cumulative effects of this process result in improved functioning and health, better lifestyle habits, changes in outlook and self-care, and a host of other lasting direct benefits and effects. Secondary effects conform to the learning model described by operant conditioning. Practice with neurofeedback training, in essence, allows the brain to witness its own patterns, and the endogenous neuromodulation facilitates enduring changes, which the brain and the environment reinforce.

At the level of neurological influence (the agency of training effect), advanced development of these techniques allows for improvement beyond the operant conditioning effect by making use of deeper neural network rhythms that show brainwave patterns at *infra-low* levels as basic as one ten thousandth of a hertz (Hz).[10] This level of brain observation has extremely powerful effects on positively modifying brain flexibility and enhancing the ability to control fight-or-flight response at the autonomic level and to heal trauma without language or restimulation.

While playing the game or watching a movie or video, we are being reinforced neurologically at the rate of approximately 3,000 "rewards" per session as our brain is being shown how to adjust its timing mechanisms to more functional and "feel good" levels. All we have to do is sit in a comfortable chair and observe the computer screen. Our job in the training process is to bear witness to our own brain activity. The process is fascinating!

But how does this exercise help us overcome challenges, symptoms, illnesses, setbacks, and the conflict that results from living in a difficult world? Read on . . .

---

10. Here frequency refers to the number of complete rhythmic cycles per second. Typically, humans measure frequencies between 0–3 Hz (sleepy waves) and 50–100 Hz (physically strenuous activity or fight-or-flight bursts). *Infra-low* activity occurs simultaneously and is more fundamental to self-regulatory functions and the brain's programming and projection of future activity. The elongated time period to complete each cycle (hours to days) allows the brain to witness patterns of biological activity otherwise unavailable to conscious observation (e.g., compare to electron microscopes facilitating observation of cell structures).

How Neurofeedback Works

The beauty of neurofeedback is that it makes a cause-and-effect relationship easily observable and accessible—as simple as noticing when a variety of elements on the screen appear and disappear, go faster or slower, or when sounds become more frequent, rhythmic, or melodic. Games can range from fast moving, stimulating, and sleek (such as car or spaceship games) to quiet and calming games (such as those with flowers, bubbles, and music).

Many games appeal easily to children's natural abilities. Because the process is nonverbal, even very young and severely impaired children can engage with them successfully. For example, in some games, geometric shapes on the screen become bigger or smaller, objects are positioned higher or lower, and sounds go on or off. Following such cues is easy and natural, since we develop the basic perceptual skills that are required by the age of two. A key feature to the efficacy of neurofeedback is that the games are interactive with the nervous system—not with logic, achievement, language, or other higher cognitive skills. I have used this training with blind people with only sound feedback and with deaf people with only visual feedback. The brain is keenly sensitive and capable of seeking information through the available channels.

The brain characteristics of critical importance involve the various brainwave frequencies (electrical cycles per second) that "carry" information from one part of the brain to another, much like radio signals carry information from transmitter towers to a radio. A natural ebb and flow in this activity is detected by the sensitive computer instrumentation. The information about preferred brainwaves is represented within the game itself, i.e., larger brainwaves may appear as a larger box or a wider bar on the screen, or they may advance a spaceship or slow it down.

Remarkably, the brain can easily figure out what is required to make the game go just as steering a wheel to the left will make a car turn in that direction. You make the game advance just by watching the screen; the brain likes continuity and naturally alters its brainwaves in order to keep the game "going."

Eventually, the brain learns and continues the key elements and subtleties. The neurofeedback software uses inhibiting thresholds that simultaneously show the brain when it is engaging in "out-of-control" activity. Eventually, you control of your brainwaves makes these changes happen on the computer screen. This improved control is what translates into more appropriate and functional behaviors in everyday living.

In EEG neurofeedback, learning occurs at a neurological level, training brain behavior that we may not feel strongly connected to or particularly responsibility for. By witnessing your own brain in action, you can watch it meander from success to struggle and back to success. The neurofeedback process teaches you about your own visible behavior while your brain is simultaneously learning about itself in a unique and replicable way. Learning accelerates and modifies behavior rapidly and efficiently.

When brain behavior is normalized, outward behavior naturally follows. Life begins to become more manageable, often with very little additional conscious effort. Brain abilities develop that translate to other life situations, because these abilities are fundamental, allowing the brain to remain calm, organized, and focused, whereas otherwise it might escalate into too much excitability or lapse into disorganization.

Role of EEG Neurofeedback in Weight Loss and Control

Overeating, mindless eating, and impulse control are influenced by our brain self-management, therefore gaining better control of brain regulation to help control behavior control, make strategic eating choices, and reduce stressful reactions that precipitate faulty eating. Neurofeedback is a valuable tool in gaining our control over our minds and bodies, using a neurophysiological basis to put us back in charge. By helping sleep, mental clarity, and emotional balance, we can better plan and implement eating habits that get our desired results.

Thought Fields and Thought Field Therapy (TFT)

Whereas neurofeedback underpins self-regulation, modulates stress reactions, and promotes the physiological aspects of appetite and satiety awareness, it will not solve eating or obesity problems by itself. Another powerful intervention that is extremely useful for eliminating cravings, self-sabotage, and the traumatic foundations that underly eating and other compulsions is Thought Field Therapy (TFT).

TFT was developed by Dr. Roger Callahan, who began this work in the 1970s and continued to expand and refine the methods and applications. He published seminal works about TFT and trained thousands of professionals in its therapeutic utilization. In my own experience working with and learning from Dr. Callahan, I saw firsthand how effective this method is, and I have used it for many decades with my own patients.

At its inception, TFT was used primarily to eliminate anxiety-based problems such as phobias and panic and various types of trauma. Over time, practitioners expanded the range of applications to effectively use TFT in the treatment of many physical ills such as headaches, digestive upsets, and body pain. Startling developments in the practical applications of TFT have included its use in Kosovo and Africa to treat war trauma and many variants of the posttraumatic stress and injury associated with violence, loss, abandonment, torture, and deprivation. TFT has wide-ranging applications for the relief of all types of negative emotions, as well as symptoms of physiological distress and psychological self-sabotage. The technique works fast with remarkable efficacy. And self-help versions of TFT are easy to use, convenient, and contribute to self-control and self-empowerment.

Numerous influences can upset internal balance and lead to improper eating. Many foods elicit biochemical compulsions and addictions, and repetitive indulgence reinforces maladaptive habits. Cravings, withdrawal, stress, varying negative emotional states, neuronal dysregulation, disrupted schedules, and other factors upset the apple cart—but the key dynamic and underlying player in these dysfunctional cycles that breaks down control is the infusion and persistence of anxiety. TFT is a powerful technique that will enable you to escape anxiety in minutes (without chemicals), thereby increasing your self-control and ability to carry out intentional adaptive choices more regularly.

Anxiety is a natural mammalian response to actual or perceived threat or the sensation or expectation of exposure or danger that is a physiological response that propels the nervous system into a fight-or-flight state. This reaction is complicated by the conscious mind's perception of high alert and the conditioned response of the cognitive mind to explain, interpret, or justify the automatic neurological reaction. People who experience high anxiety associate this uncomfortable feeling with distressing thoughts, images, or memories. The thoughts and feelings become intertwined, usually in such a way that the anxious person often believes that the thoughts are what is causing the anxiety. But cognitive thoughts do not *cause* anxiety (although they may accompany, reinforce, and harmonize with physiological anxiety). The physiological and visceral response comes first, habitually triggering the mind's *narrative* to explain, interpret, and justify the anxious experience.

The interconnection between visceral neurological/emotional states and thoughts that accompany them constructs a *negative thought field*. Such formations tend to keep the connections bound together, almost like a chemical reaction. When this state endures, the negative thought field binds the negative emotion (anxiety) regardless of its origination.

Though a "thought field" may seem like an abstract concept, thought fields can be measured physiologically, subjectively, and empirically. Negative thought fields, once identified, can be *eliminated* by TFT. Treatment with TFT, or its advanced version called *Voice Technology* (*VT*), collapses the structure of negative thought fields by eliminating the *perturbations* (disruptions in the energy flow) that bind the negative thoughts and feelings, thus rapidly eliminating the distress.

Although negative emotions are a normal part of our makeup, all too often negativity drives our behavior and attitudes, even without our realizing how pivotal these emotions are in promoting or interfering with our capacity to live intact. Rampant negative emotions can disable or paralyze the psychological flexibility we require to engage alternate responses, colluding with our mind's negative and justifying narrative and keeping us stuck.

When negative thought fields are eliminated, the result is a complete absence of the previous (just before treatment) experiences of anxiety, trauma, and other negative emotions. In some cases, only one or a few treatments result in the prolonged absence of the treated negative emotions. With phobias in particular, we can accurately conclude that the disturbance is *cured*. Persistent and chronic anxiety is more complicated and requires a broader understanding and approach that is found in TFT.

Thought Field Therapy (TFT) Terms

Thought Field Therapy. A treatment for psychological disturbances that provides a *code* that, when applied to a psychological problem on which the individual is focusing, eliminates *perturbations* in the thought field that is the fundamental cause of all negative emotions.

Thought field. A *field* is an invisible, nonmaterial structure in space that has an effect upon matter. A *thought field* is a connection between cognitive awareness and emotions that *generates a field that may contain perturbations.*

Perturbation: Perturbations are the physiological, neurological, hormonal, chemical, and cognitive events that result in the experience of specific negative emotions.

Cure. The cure of a health problem is the elimination of all subjective experience of distress and symptoms associated with it.[11] In TFT, a cure is brought about by eliminating perturbations in the thought field.

Using Thought Field Therapy

Thought Field Therapy (TFT) is a powerful yet simple treatment for dealing with psychological disturbances by manipulating how energy flows in the body. TFT does not require any equipment, and a therapist is not needed to carry out many parts of the treatment. Although TFT can be self-administered with quick and effective results, some people do not respond as well to self-treatment or may prefer working with a therapist.

When applied to a psychological problem a person is experiencing, TFT eliminates perturbations in the thought field that are the fundamental cause of negative emotions—a process that is similar to reprogramming a computer task by providing or revising computer codes. By finger tapping on specific energy points in a particular code sequence, the TFT process

---

11. In psychological treatment and research, a measure of subjective distress that is often used is a rating scale called a SUD (subjective unit of distress), whereby a person rates their distress on a scale of 1–10, where 10 is the most distress conceivable and 1 represents no distress or symptom.

causes these perturbations to collapse, and renders them inactive. To fathom how and why TFT works, we must remember that nature uses various codes to operate, signal, and modify the world. Humans use codes, consciously and biologically, in many ways.

Nature's Codes

Nature overflows with secrets and mysteries contained in environmental and biological codes. Examples include barometric pressure that indicates when it is likely to rain, cramping or bloating that indicate when a menstrual period is coming, and fatigue and stress that signal the need to rest, retreat, and recover.

From DNA to language, symbols, and relationships, the world is embedded with information about how life unfolds. Managing life requires the detection, translation, and enactment of the codes that encapsulate this information. We use codes for analyzing and synthesizing data, formulating concepts and logic, testing hypotheses, evaluating options, and generalizing from our individual and collective experiences the characteristics, resources, and courses of action that help us survive and live better.

Codes sum up the rules and messages about these processes. For example, when driving, we respond to traffic lights at an intersection. We use social codes to indicate our receptivity and availability, and we react to the green/red light messages that tell whether it is okay to proceed on a course. We are attuned to people's facial expressions that convey whether to advance, back off, or wait. Codes communicate when the airplane bathroom is vacant, the degree to which a social gesture is welcome, when a boundary has been violated, and even when a partner might be interested in sex. Formally or informally taught cognitive codes that are reflected in expressive language, grammatical conventions, spelling rules, mathematics, and economic principles allow us to communicate our ideas and exchange goods and services.

Codes for Identification, Communication, and Brain Function

Codes embed information akin to shorthand methods for abbreviating, storing, and communicating information—like our Social Security number and the many PIN (personal identification number) codes and passwords we create to protect and access private information. Though we may not think of it this way, information we hear or see is also coded. For example, the English language contains twenty-six letters that can be combined to form words, sentences, and limitless ideas. When we read or listen to information, we decode the words in accordance with accepted rules of phonetics, pronunciation, and grammar. If we understand what the decoded words mean, we can process and assimilate the encoded information. If the information is represented in numbers (e.g., the balance of our checking account or in computer language) and we've mastered the meaning of these number codes, we are then able to respond accordingly.

Biological data can be decoded, and by breaking the codes, beneficial alterations in human response patterns can be achieved. TFT allows such code "replacements" to occur in our body and brain by replacing harmful or distressing codes with those that are beneficial and healing. For many, this is a radical concept to consider: that the body and mind store coded information that keeps emotional and physical problems in place, and that by decoding and reprogramming this information, negative feelings and problems can be alleviated, typically within minutes.

Think of the function of the codes that our body stores as a kind of emotional alarm system. The alarm is set within us by reactions we have to traumas, upsets, and even to foods and medicines. TFT deactivates the internal alarm and offsets the signals that trigger the alarms. This is accomplished by tapping with our fingers on specifically identified points on our body in a specific order. The tapping, via meridian points and pathways, sends energy signals throughout our nervous system that disrupt the perturbations that are causing the distress. They essentially reset our system back to "normal" for the particular problem that was upsetting us.

To grasp the concept of how pressing with our fingertips can create so much impact, think of a garage door opener. Or better yet, think of how tapping several numbers into a phone can send specific messages over a great distance with great speed and impact. Once the negative emotional charge is removed, we can think clearly about the problem, but it will no longer bother us at all. *Poof!*

An interesting and common phenomenon that often occurs after a rapid TFT treatment that totally eliminates the problem, is when the treated person says, "I can't think about it anymore." The person is really saying, "When I think about it, it doesn't bother me."

In general, tapping on meridian points can have a beneficial effect. Several "look-alike" tapping treatments claim efficacy, and some may work to a certain degree; but the detection of the disruptive codes and application of the functional codes are the real secrets to TFT's astounding and consistent success. Curative codes elicited through TFT's causal diagnostic procedure permitted the development of the TFT algorithms—shortcuts or general tapping recipes that have emerged over time as common tapping sequences. They can be self-administered while thinking of the problem and are often effective in eliminating the problem.

More About Perturbations

The fundamental cause of emotional distress, including anxiety and cravings, is the phenomenon of perturbation in the thought field. This specific type of information that resides in the thought field contains the instructions for triggering and thus generating the chemical and neurological events that lead to what we call negative or disturbing emotions. Many of these perturbations are inherited, and some are established during the lifetime of the individual. Regardless of the origin, TFT can eliminate these negative emotions at their fundamental source.

The basic premise of TFT is that the perturbations in the thought field precede and generate these chemical and cognitive events. Chemical events in the human body will ultimately result in negative emotions as well as associated cognitive thoughts and related neurological activity. These perturbations that form the fundamental and basic cause of all disturbed or negative emotions are subsumed and rendered inoperative with successful TFT treatment. The successful therapeutic treatment of the perturbation eliminates the chemical and cognitive consequences. The perturbation is the basic causal factor and the chemistry and cognition are considered secondary and tertiary.

Proof of this phenomenon exists at physiological *and* psychological levels. At the physiological level, research shows that *heart rate variability*

(HRV) improves dramatically after TFT treatment.[12] For this reason, I especially recommend TFT treatment to anyone with a history of heart problems.

At the psychological level, a person's narrative changes dramatically after treatment. Because patients in distress routinely feel impelled to repeat their description of symptoms and all the negative ramifications, I ask my patients to do the TFT treatment first, and I agree to listen to their story for as long as they want afterward. But almost always after a TFT treatment of just a few minutes, the patient has no story left to tell—the symptoms that were driving the story (which seemed very real and rooted in external circumstances) have essentially *disappeared*.

How Can This Possibly Happen Within Minutes?

Good question!

Let's review some realities we usually take for granted and compare their relevance to feeling well. Take body temperature, for example. We are warm-blooded animals who must maintain body temperature within a relatively narrow range in order to function. When body temperature fluctuates more than a few degrees, we become symptomatic (chills, fever), and we can become at risk for survival. Fortunately, the human body has built-in mechanisms for maintaining and regulating body temperature, as it does for many other functions, including "emotional temperature."

When body temperature is controlled, it is difficult to feel or even imagine a physical threat from heat or cold. However, step outside in subzero temperatures or sit in a bath that is too hot, and you will know firsthand the experience of responding rapidly to environmental changes with negative feelings. However, the reverse—experiencing rapid changes in positive feelings—is also possible, and yet taken for granted.

---

12. Heart rate variability (HRV) is a primary indicator of the body's resources to survive and adapt to internal and external challenges. Poor HRV is associated with morbidity and premorbid disease conditions. HRV is one of the most researched variables in medicine. Until recently, scientists did not have methods of improving HRV significantly and rapidly. My colleagues and I have shown dramatic improvements in HRV after a single TFT session (Pignotti and Steinberg, 2001).

Physical examples that illustrate this principle provide relevance to emotional healing. When you come in from the cold or remove the source of the heat, your body quickly acclimates back to its accustomed range of comfortable operation. Unless you were exposed to the point of actual physical injury (burns, frostbite, or hypothermia), you recover relatively quickly, usually within minutes. Given the degree of threat posed by "the elements," this rapid recovery might seem surprising—yet we take it for granted because temperature acclimatization is within our experience and happens automatically and consistently.

Physical illness also illustrates the self-healing/self-regulating phenomenon. Most have experienced the massive discomfort that accompanies a high fever as our bodily defenses mobilize to contain the offending microbes when stricken by a virus such as a "twenty-four-hour flu." The critical period when the fever "breaks" is followed by a rapid acceleration in recovery, and a noticeable relief or "feeling better," and we take for granted that returning to normalcy will happen relatively quickly.

With rare exceptions, people don't live with high fevers for very long. The body's immune system must overcome and contain the invading pathogens. Our white blood cells surround foreign organisms to encapsulate pathogens and prevent them from multiplying and taking over our bodies. This isolation process usually happens automatically (although we can take steps to facilitate the process), whether or not we intellectually comprehend the ever-vigilant, self-healing phenomenon operating within our body. Similarly, nature has encoded mechanisms within us to absorb, fight, and mitigate emotional and psychological invasions. To ensure survival, nature insists that we subdue threat, lest it overpower and defeat us.

The psychologically programmed mechanism that reduces emotional threats isolates them by tucking them away (encoding them) into specific energy and nervous system disruptions that are much less of a threat to the entire organism. These isolated and specific disruptions (perturbations) are activated by thought fields—that emotional discomfort aroused when a person thinks about something connected to the original perturbation. Thoughts connected with the "encoded" threat are experienced as the symptoms of a psychological problem. TFT is an ideally suited and simple tool for treating those symptoms—effectively reprogramming the mechanism to override the perturbations.

TFT in Practice

TFT is done by finger tapping on specific meridian points or energy points, on the upper body when experiencing the negative emotion or urge you want to eliminate. The same meridian points are used in acupuncture treatment. Tapping can be done with either hand. Self-tapping is convenient and allows for autonomy and self-sufficiency. But having another person administer tapping is fine as well.

The effectiveness is derived from energy put into the body by the tapping. When applied at the appropriate junctures in the correct sequences, the tapping *transduces* (converts and sends) slight physical/kinesthetic energy signals to the brain and nervous system to alters and reprogram the linkages between thoughts and feelings. This eliminates the negative emotions and empowers behavioral change.

The same concept is easy to recognize in its application to many other simple operations we take for granted. The programming of an alarm is similar, where tapping in the appropriate code disengages the alarm. Certain eye movements as well as humming may also be used at some points in the process.

When the mind and body are in distress, a thought field is connected to a negative emotional state (alarm), and the appropriate tapping breaks the connection with the embedded code that set created the disturbance (alarm) in the first place. The process of decoding any disturbance caused by perturbations comprises the diagnostic aspects of TFT, which applies our body's natural wisdom to unlock the codes that affect our conscious and subconscious thoughts, feelings, and behavioral motivations to achieve relief.

Step-by-Step Instruction for Self-Help through Algorithms

In this example, we use anxiety and cravings (or addictive urges) as the negative emotion we want to eliminate. Cravings and addictive urges span

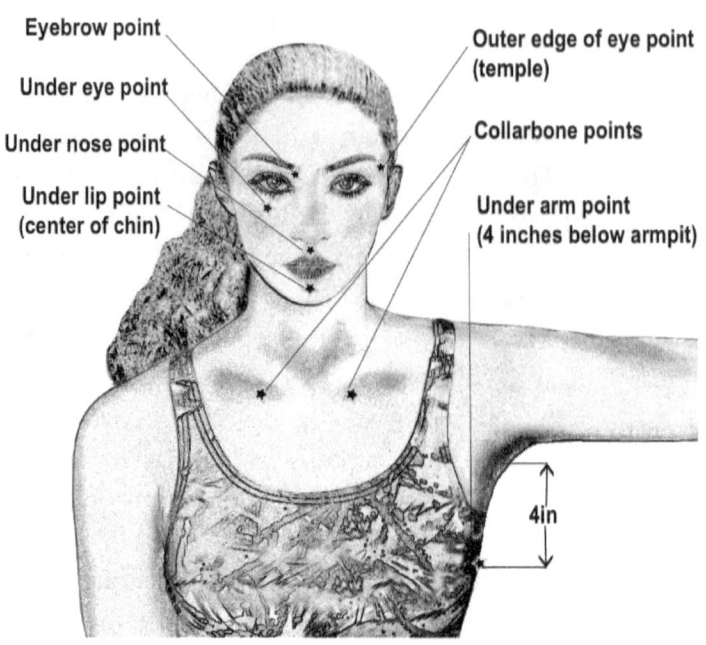

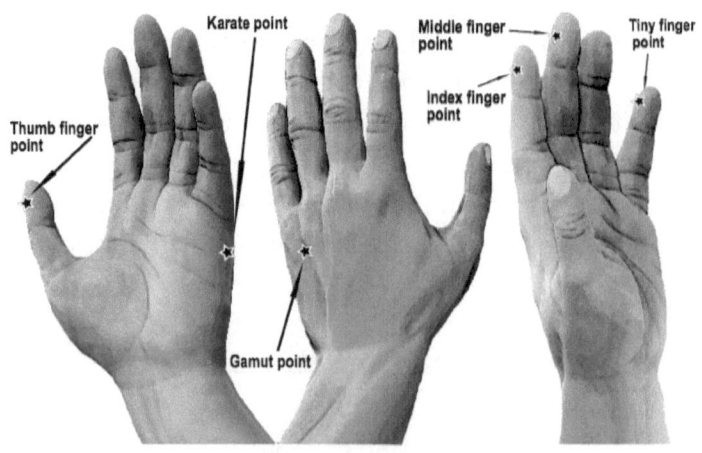

a spectrum of severity and frequency, but here we are addressing urges and cravings we prefer not to have. Anxiety is a fundamental negative emotion that drives much of uncomfortable narratives and problematic behaviors. Tapping points are shown in the diagram.

Review all the steps to get a sense of the process. For the first treatment, wait until your anxiety or urge is quite high to noticeably experience the dramatic power of the treatment. Repeat treatments any time you are aware of any anxiety or an unwanted urge or craving.

1. **Rate your anxiety/urge.**
   Rate and write down the degree of your current urge on a 10-point scale from 1 (no anxiety/urge at all) to 10 (the anxiety/urge is highest).

2. **Treat the urge.**
   Take the first two fingers of either hand and tap underneath one of your eyes (See diagram) solidly and firmly 15X (do not hurt yourself).
   Tap the collarbone point 15X.
   Tap the underarm point located four inches below your armpit 15X.
   Tap the collarbone point again 15X.

If your anxiety/urge remains the same after these treatments, a corrective procedure called psychological reversal (PR) is useful. If you do the corrective procedure (shown after the sequence) and tap under your eyes again, you should notice a definite (not subtle) and clear reduction in your anxiety/addictive urge. Otherwise continue with the nine-gamut (energy point) treatment sequence

The Nine-Gamut Treatment Sequence
The nine-gamut treatment will result in further reducing the anxiety or urge. Continue to think of your urge and tap solidly (with two fingers) the gamut spot on the back of your hand behind and between the little finger knuckle and the ring finger knuckle on the back of your hand. (See

diagram) It doesn't matter which hand you use, but many prefer to tap with the dominant hand on the back of the nondominant hand. Keep your head straight with your nose pointed ahead while doing this treatment.

Tap about 5X for each of the nine gamut positions, while continuing to think of your anxiety or addictive urge. This step includes eye movements.

While tapping gamut spot on back of hand, do the following:

1. Close your eyes.
2. Open your eyes.
3. Point your eyes down and to the right.
4. Point your eyes down and to the left.
5. Whirl your eyes around in a circle.
6. Whirl your eyes around in the opposite direction.
7. Rest your eyes, and hum any tune—more than just one note (for about 5 seconds).
8. Count aloud 1–5.
9. Hum again (important).

Repeat the 9 gamut tapping sequence under the eyes, collarbone point, under arm, and collarbone point while you think of any remaining urge.

At this point, the urge or interest in your particular anxiety or addiction will likely be completely gone. If you try to resurrect your targeted urge, you probably won't able to do so. Remember how easy it was to fall into engaging in your anxiety/addictive urge. But this too should have no effect on you, because you have, at least temporarily, eliminated your stress in these areas. Observe how relaxed you feel, the natural relaxation brought on by the removal of an underlying problem. This is normal and healthy, not false and destructive.

Tapping correctly treats the underlying problem causing the anxiety or addictive urge. Many problems amenable to TFT require only one treatment, but addictive urges tend to recur. With the ease and expediency of self-treatment, it is simple and practical to keep treating the anxiety/urge as often as needed.

After successful TFT treatment, any recurrence of anxiety/urges or problem is usually due to an *individual energy toxin* (IET). Toxins are a critically important issue for many people and especially for those en-meshed in negative addictive cycles. Toxins often induce a psychological reversal that has the effect of "undoing" or reversing a previously success-ful treatment and also of interfering or blocking the progress of an incip-ient treatment. Aside from its impact upon TFT treatments, the effect of psychological reversal is a major factor in many other treatment protocols and can undermine desired goal-oriented motivational states.

Fortunately such psychological reversal (PR) can be corrected.

How to Correct Psychological Reversal (PR)

A psychological reversal exists when a person professes a desire to achieve a specific goal, but the person's actions and major motivation, as well as their results, appear to be contrary to the professed goal. The person may appear to be striving to achieve (in the *specifically reversed* area), but will instead be significantly or subtly and unintentionally sabotaging the effort.

Psychological reversal can be tested when a person is attuned to a targeted thought field—an invisible, intangible structure in space that has an effect upon matter—the connection between cognitive awareness and emotions that generates it. For a phobic person, perhaps the thought of getting on an airplane or confronting an insect may generate an intense negative reaction. The thought generates the field that contains distur-bances responsible for the negative emotional reactions.

Testing for the reversal is part of the TFT diagnostic routine that is administered by professionally trained TFT practitioners, and the result is easily determined in a matter of seconds. Because TFT treatment works so rapidly, psychological reversals are easy to address as well. A reversal can be seen in physiology and muscle strength/weakness that people ex-perience when stressed. Lie detection methods measure stress indicators such as heart rate, blood pressure, respiration rate, and GSR (galvanic skin response).

Psychological reversal can be specialized, only affecting certain areas of one's life; or less commonly, it can be wide-reaching and affect much of one's life in a negative way. The incidence of massive reversal is higher in people who have struggled with severe anxiety and addictions or other psychological problems for a long time.

Psychological reversals must be corrected for successful treatment progression and to counter self-sabotaging behavior. Corrections involve specific tapping on the side of the hand or under the nose, depending upon when the reversals occur in the treatment sequence.

When a person thinks about their aspirations or positive goals, the feelings involved should be strength and health—not weakness and sickness. But some seemingly highly motivated individuals do not succeed, no matter what program, method of treatment, coaching technique, or educational procedure is used. Many clinicians have noted that certain patients, even while the patient is actively seeking help, seem to *want* to be ill, or *want* to be disturbed, or even die. (Freud postulated a death instinct.) Others have suggested that most neurotics are self-sabotaging and self-defeating. Some traditional psychoanalytic constructs find parallels with modern neurophysiological findings.

The will, or control over oneself, is definitely limited in a reversed state. The choices available are restricted to negative ones, and the thoughts and ideas tend to have a negative slant. In a severe state of psychological reversal, there is strong resistance to trying or doing the recommended procedures, treatments, or lifestyle changes that would aid in relief of the affliction or symptoms. A person in a state of psychological reversal is unable to respond favorably to an otherwise effective treatment. However, if the reversal is corrected, the person will respond to an effective treatment.

The incidence of psychological reversal varies according to the specific problem. For example, anxiety and phobic problems have a 40–50 percent reversal incidence. Almost half of phobic problems may be blocked from getting completely better. Once the TFT treatment for psychological reversal was discovered, the success rate for treating phobias and anxiety immediately increased dramatically after the simple and fast correction for psychological reversal was administered. The incidence of psychological reversal is higher among addicts than for other groups.

The phenomenon of psychological reversal is measurable; its effects are predictable, regular, and scientifically lawful. TFT brings good news even to the most negatively suffering people. TFT treatment for psychological reversal is simple. The subject must tap on the side of the hand (PR spot) or tap under the nose (See figure) when attuned to the thought in the treatment sequence. These "subconscious" obstacles can be fixed *in seconds* with specific sequential taps. Correcting psychological reversals becomes more targeted and effective when the therapist is trained in TFT diagnostic methods.

The Apex Problem

Many people are familiar with "overthinking" a situation, a mind game of wrong thinking that usually presents as dismissiveness. This is known as the *apex problem*. For many, because TFT works so rapidly (which seems illogical), the mind will make things up in order to explain the dissonance with the person's assumptions. Anyone who does TFT regularly with others is certain to encounter this phenomenon and needs to understand what is happening.

The term "apex problem" is borrowed from Callahan (2002) who cites Koestler (1967), referring to the operation of the mind at its peak (or apex). The commonly observed fact by clinicians is that many patients who receive TFT treatment for *any* particular problem will accurately report the expected and predicted improvement, but will typically *not* credit the treatment for the improvement. They suggest explanations such as placebo, suggestion, distraction, etc.

This phenomenon has basic scientific relevance in that its frequent occurrence leads to a prediction that recipients of treatment may not credit the treatment for the dramatic change of state they report after the treatment—and that many who are successfully treated will invent other explanations in order to avoid the obvious fact of the role of the treatment. It seems that in order to credit this surprisingly effective treatment, some people diminish cognitive dissonance (with logic) by considering the treatment as a "miracle." Some successfully treated individuals actually say, "It was a miracle!"

TFT does sometimes appear as a kind of miracle (something amazing, extraordinary, and unexpected, seemingly contrary to the laws of nature). However, TFT works according to the laws of nature, including scientific laws. Despite its replicable efficacy, the people who have trouble accommodating the seemingly nonlinear effects will, after successful treatment, either deny the problem they had before the treatment or minimize it; or they will acknowledge that they feel better, but attribute the change to some explanation other than the treatment.

When they think about the problem that previously caused a severe emotional reaction, they no longer feel any distress or preoccupation about it. Patients may report some version of, "You distracted me from thinking about the problem with that tapping," or "I just can't think about it right now." Patients are far less likely to wonder about the possible curative role of their surgery, just as addicts may ignore the role of their successful rehabilitation therapy.

In his "split-brain" experiments, neuroscientist Michael S. Gazzaniga discovered that the language aspect of the left brain will invent and create "explanations" for phenomena that are introduced to the nonverbal right brain and not known to the left.[13] However, the left brain, observing the behavior, will compulsively "explain" what is taking place, even though there is no basis in fact for the "explanation." It is purely irrelevant invention.

Another striking example of the apex problem is with hypnosis—when a subject is given a posthypnotic suggestion with amnesia. Subjects may offer irrelevant "explanations" for their behavior because the behavior seems strange to them. The speed and stunning effectiveness of TFT treatment seems to generate the apex problem mostly in those vulnerable to it. Since nothing the person has previously known accounts for the dramatic result, many subjects and observers will compulsively *tell* (not ask) why the change took place (i.e., placebo effect, hypnosis, or distraction). That the explainer has never witnessed similar demonstrations of the power of placebo, hypnosis, or distraction appears to carry little weight.

Prior explanations before treatment appear to have little effect upon reducing the apex problem. Perhaps this issue will subside further as TFT and its results become more generally known and recognized.

In addiction treatment, the mind is confronted with a phenomenon it can't comprehend, i.e., immediate successful treatment; so the logical "left brain," in Gazzaniga's terms, begins inventing (irrelevant) explanations even though, in the addiction treatment, the brain's hemispheres are intact,

---

13. Gazzaniga, M. 1985. *The Social Brain*, NY: Basic Books.

and there is no hypnosis nor induced amnesia. The compulsion to invent familiar and effortless explanation appears to override critical thinking.

This same phenomenon probably occurs in most people at times in life, and the commonplace nature of this interesting phenomenon will be obvious to anyone using TFT regularly.

How Long Do Treatment Results Last?

The endurance of the treatment for an addictive urge, anxiety, or other negative emotion varies from person to person and even for the same person at different times. In my experience administering thousands of treatments mostly using Voice Technology, this highest level of TFT has a success rate of 97 percent for any single treatment. About 80 percent of the people I treat have required one or two treatments to experience successful results that last indefinitely. The other 20 percent have recurrences due mostly to toxins (described earlier). Traumas and phobias are among the conditions that Voice Technology with TFT treatment successfully treats with enduring results. Addictions and obsessive-compulsive disorders typically require repeated treatment.

The severity of the problem is not an accurate predictor of TFT success. One might think that traumas such as abuse, sexual molestation, war horrors, loss of a loved one, etc., would be so deeply entrenched that little could relieve, much less eliminate these sufferings. Yet using Voice Technology TFT, I have routinely eliminated issues such as these in a single treatment.

Examples:

- ✓ A woman who lost her husband and son in a car accident that she survived. She had been depressed by this trauma for nine years.
- ✓ Multiple cases of sexual molestation and childhood abuse.
- ✓ People suffering flashbacks from war experiences.
- ✓ Survivors of Nazi concentration camps.
- ✓ A man traumatized and plagued by an incident that occurred a half-century ago.

I do not suggest that TFT can undo the horrible realities that people endure. I am simply stating unequivocally, and with solid proof, that the emotional *sting* of these traumatic experiences can be removed *completely* within minutes. The success and endurance experienced with TFT depends on a number of factors:

- The degree of psychological reversal.
- One's sensitivity to toxins.
- Correct implementation of the procedures and persistence in repetition when necessary.
- One's general health.
- The nature (not severity) of the problem being treated.

Please note that one's *belief* in the efficacy of the treatment is not listed as a factor in predictive success. This is because *it does not matter*. Like an antibiotic, TFT will either work or it won't, *irrespective of one's beliefs*. One simply has to administer it.

Self-help treatment is not as effective as professional treatment for more complex cases. However, self-help treatment has the advantages of being free, convenient, and private—and often works splendidly. So why not try it?

TFT has no negative side effects. The only potential downside to self-help TFT treatment is that if you don't experience satisfactory results quickly, you may give up, dismiss TFT, and pass up an extremely valuable tool for living intact, simply because you didn't get significant relief the first or second time. For this reason, I suggest contacting a professional when a self-administered procedure does not appear to be working. Be aware of how TFT works, how it differs in practice and theory from conventional treatments, and how the apex problem can lead you astray.

The vast majority of people will experience profound calmness and significant reduction in anxiety, urges, and cravings the first and every time they use the TFT algorithms. A small number of people can do just one urge-reduction treatment and never have a further desire for their addictive substance. This, alas, is a rare response, but it does happen.

For most people, cravings will return at the first sign of stress, and it is imperative to repeat the treatment each time an urge arises. Frequency of treatment depends upon the degree of stress. Keep in mind that repeated treatments are not wasted—rather, each administration of the procedure treats the underlying cause of the addiction problem. Since the underlying problem is addressed and treated (rather than being masked as with tranquilizers), repeated treatments may eventually eliminate it completely.

The resurfacing of negative emotions, once handily treated, often indicates other thought fields that need treatment because, aside from toxins and psychological reversal, many problems are undergirded by negative emotions that contain multiple thought fields. A skilled TFT practitioner is adept at helping patients identify and target relevant perturbed thought fields.

The Three Levels of TFT Treatment

Algorithms are "summary recipes" for administering TFT that have resulted from applying the commonalities of thousands of individually diagnosed perturbation sequences. Algorithms are what nonprofessionals typically use to treat themselves (finger tapping, etc.).

Causal diagnosis is the objective scientific procedure of identifying perturbations (specific to particular thought fields) and determining which tapping points and in what order will be most effective in *collapsing* the perturbations—that is, decoding or deprogramming the thought field so that the perturbations causing the disturbance are no longer active. Causal diagnosis involves a combination of helping the patient *attune* the thought field and then using variations of applied kinesiology (muscle testing) to identify the active perturbations. The practitioner typically does this by "testing" various points on the patient's body.

Voice Technology (**VT**) is the practice of diagnosing the points through information provided by the patient's voice. This most-advanced level of TFT offers a number of advantages including the obvious expediency of treating someone effectively by phone. VT is quicker and often more precise in treating patients with greater complexity or long strings of perturbations and is expedient in the identification of toxins that may cause psychological reversals and interfere with treatment. Toxic substances that cause a psychological reversal, and may block or reverse the effects of successful treatment, typically include various foods, toiletries, aromas, and supplements that act are harmful to a percentage of people. For many, the sustained positive effects of treatments and better health require the identification of and abstention from toxins.

Nature encodes the sources of distress and their solutions within our bodies and minds. Because of nature's recapitulation and signaling system, the human voice indicates with precision the causes of emotional and physical disturbance and can be used in tandem with TFT to eliminate the source and symptoms in minutes.

Applications of TFT Treatment

TFT is useful for eliminating a wide array of problems. By eliminating negative emotions with consistency, a new world unfolds—a world of personal freedom in which a person can set their mind to achieve some goal, identify the emotional traps that so heavily and surreptitiously disrupt their well-being and impede their purposefully desired behavior, and attain one goal after another as they progress on to a better life, away from the shackles of anxiety and its cohorts.

A partial list of negative emotions TFT can eliminate:

Anxiety	Stress	Guilt	Cravings
Depression	Overwhelm	Hopelessness	Emotional/behavioral overreaction
Frustration	Irritation	Disgust	Jealousy/lovesickness
Anger	Fear	Rejection	Worry

TFT with Eating and Weight Issues

TFT applications are many and varied and is also effective when self-administered. Its utility in eating and managing weight center around the control of emotions through the rapid elimination of the stress and distress that often lead to impulsive or poor eating for relief. Principal uses of TFT are to:

- Eliminate negative emotions.
- Eliminate cravings.
- Correct psychological reversals that sabotage good intentions and plans.

Those having difficulty implementing the techniques or who may need more advanced intervention can easily contact a clinician (like me) who can provide help by phone using Voice Technology.

The Need for Physiological and Emotional Control

Engaging in professional help requires an investment of effort, time, and expense. Fortunately, TFT can be learned and self-administered, and its more advanced and rapidly effective version—Voice Technology—can be done by phone. EEG neurofeedback typically requires in-office professional treatment. However, with experienced supervision and using the proper equipment, neurofeedback can also be done at home. Caution: be wary of inexpensive devices available online that usually don't provide adequate results and safeguards for brain health.

Food issues, eating habits, and weight-control issues comprise a complicated and interrelated mélange of brain and gut connections, metabolic functions, behavioral habits, and physiological and emotional regulation. Notwithstanding nutritional realities and the harmful ways many foods can affect us negatively, our efforts to control eating, weight, and our overall relationship with food and our body are highly influenced by the success we have with physiological and emotional regulation and the management and dispatch of stress and negative emotions. This is why I include EEG neurofeedback and TFT as integral parts of my recommended and most successful weight control program.

CHAPTER 12

Behavior Modification

Change What You Do

Along with the biological drives and mechanisms that influence how we feel and act, self-control and managing behaviors that congeal into habits are of paramount concern in many areas of functioning, including eating.

So what are the elements and rules that control and predict our behaviors?

How can we take charge of what we do, and move toward desired goals?

How do we change habits and eliminate undesirable behaviors?

Eating Behavior Modification

Along with the neurophysiological and biochemical methods for controlling blood sugar, appetite, and brain-gut relationships, some behavior modification basics can be effectively applied to reprogram and control our eating habits to achieve weight control and eating goals, and be healthier.

Behavior modification refers to the theory and implementation of scientific principles that govern the ways behaviors increase or decrease, and strengthen or weaken, in accord with *contingencies*. Contingencies are if-then dependencies that establish cause-and-effect relationships between stimuli (antecedents) and their outcomes (consequences).

Originally developed and codified by B.F. Skinner, behavior modification principles govern the rules and effects of learning theory that are essentially pragmatic (without regard to desire or intention). Skinner used the term "black box" to refer to internal mind processes such as thoughts and feelings that are not directly observable in the programmable and predictable outcomes of stimulus and response contingencies. Although thoughts and feelings are also behaviors that can be modified through tangible intervention, the internal dynamics in human and animal motivation are directly attributable to control of the relationships and schedules governing stimuli and responses.

The empirical application of behavioral psychology, called behaviorism, is regarded by some as using manipulative control techniques without regard for feelings or values. But this refined technology does not exclude or preclude consciousness, morals, or ethics; it focuses scientifically on learning theory that explains, governs, and predicts how we learn and how we form and release habits.

I have used behavior modification techniques consciously and strategically in my work and life since my first introductory psychology course where we trained rats in to press a bar in their cages to deliver food and/or to avoid electric shocks. Note that *punishment* is a behavioral technique used to diminish behaviors. If, when, and how punishment is used are certainly matters of ethical concerns aside from the scientific efficacy.

Learning and Habits

Learning theory refers to a comprehensive array of scientific principles that explain and govern how we acquire, perceive, and integrate new information to form behaviors and habits. Habits are formed through repetition and practice. They may be intentional and/or desirable, or they may form without our intention or focus simply through associations between an antecedent (stimulus preceding a response) and consequences (the observable and measurable effect on an outcome tied to its antecedent).

Stimulus and response pairings happen regularly throughout our daily lives. Some are consciously directed, while others simply occur by proximity or association that, through repetition, strengthens the behavior or the probability that it will reoccur. For example, dog learns to sit when rewarded with food and praise, eventually transferring this behavior to respond to a verbal command. We behave in certain ways and work for "rewards" because we know through association and experience that certain endeavors will deliver "payoffs" that keep us interested and motivated.

When behaviors are formed and strengthened through association and repetition, we say the behaviors have been reinforced. Yelling, nail-biting, smoking, and overeating are examples of maladaptive habits that become strong and *resistant to extinction* (hard to break). The persistence of behaviors and habits conforms to predictable patterns of reinforcement that shape and strengthen behavior according to "schedules," which entail the manner and timing that determine the delivery of reinforcement.

Mental Fitness: Adaptive and Maladaptive Responses

For the purpose of evaluating and potentially changing behaviors, we classify them in two basic categories: adaptive and maladaptive. Adaptive responses (behaviors) are productive and consistent with our intention and desire for responses that lead to favorable outcomes and contribute to our goals. Gaining control of our habits, by modifying our adaptive and maladaptive behaviors, allows us to develop better mental fitness. The essence of mental fitness is the juxtaposition and balancing of two necessary and interactive components, 1) building and increasing adaptive responses, and 2) reducing and eliminating maladaptive responses.

Consider *fitness* as the ability to do work. As we become more mentally fit, our brain improves in:

- *strength*, the capacity to meet workloads and challenges;
- *endurance*, the ability to sustain performance;
- *flexibility*, the ability to modify approach according to changing conditions, needs, and requirements; and
- *resilience*, the recovery time from exertion, output, stress, and fatigue.

By becoming more mentally fit, we gain better control over our moods and body awareness, and we improve ways to harness our eating habits. The model of mental fitness, comprised of increasing adaptive responses and eliminating maladaptive responses, is a simple template for better understanding the ways we form and relinquish habits.

Behavioral learning theory principles govern how behaviors are acquired and strengthened, how habits are formed, and how behaviors are decreased or eliminated. The basic structure of behavioral acquisition and maintenances revolves around this *reinforcement* principle. We say that a behavior (conscious, intentional, or otherwise) has been reinforced when it *maintains or increases* in *frequency, intensity, or duration*.

How Reinforcement Works

We are all creatures of habit. The formation of habits occurs through strengthening or encouragement of behaviors contingent upon consequences that raise the likelihood that those behaviors will reoccur. The conditioning process (repeated reinforcement) that shapes behaviors is a two-way street: we can intentionally repeat specific behaviors with the goal of reinforcing them and forming desirable, productive habit behaviors that become automatic. Behaviors that get inadvertently or repeatedly reinforced form habits even without our conscious intention.

Habits require *practice*—and practice occurs through repetition, or *increased frequency*. Many undesirable habits are inadvertently reinforced and thereby strengthened, because they occur frequently and garner attention. Think of the disruptive child who elicits attention by constantly misbehaving, a classic example of behavior occurring often enough to sustain a robust, hard-to-break behavior. In this case, heightened frequency becomes a disadvantage.

The same principles govern eating behaviors. When we establish certain patterns of eating through repetition, our body and brain soon signal that reaching for those foods at accustomed times is necessary. The more we do so, the stronger the desire or craving. Patterns of eating combine with the biochemistry of our gut and blood sugar fluctuations to create hard-to-resist compulsions.

Though putting food into our mouth is a volitional and conscious action (despite the "mindless" eating), we are often conditioned to hunger for and capitulate to snacking or eating poorly by the effects of the reinforcement schedules we have created. When every instance of a response is reinforced, the schedule is called *continuous reinforcement*. The advantage to continuous reinforcement is that it can also facilitate the shaping of new and better behaviors, making it easy to learn new things. But continuous reinforcement is not efficient or economical. So nature provides *intermittent* reinforcement schedules that require less energy and preserve more economy and efficiency in order to maintain learned behaviors. They only reinforce *some* instances of the behavior, but not others. Intermittent schedules are useful and efficient for maintaining behaviors (but not as good for initiating or learning new behaviors).

Both types of schedules are needed. When we learn new things, we need the encouragement and practice to cement the new behavior into our repertoire (continuous reinforcement); but once the behavior is established, we only need occasional (intermittent) reinforcement to maintain the behaviors and cause them to be resistant to extinction. We have all learned thousands upon thousands of behaviors in this way—from academic skills to preparing food, driving a car, maintaining old friendships, etc.

How Reinforcement Schedules Condition Eating

We respond to cues based upon our previous patterns of behavior. If you tend to eat in response to stress, then stressful experiences (even minor ones) will trigger you to eat. If you are accustomed to eating when you sit down to watch TV, this too will signal you to eat. Even walking into your home can signal you to reach for food. These associations have been conditioned first on continuous reinforcement schedules (how you built the habit) and then on intermittent reinforcement schedules, meaning that even if you interrupt the associated behavior and trigger, the habit will resume again because it has been strengthened over time. The resilience of these habits can find us eating just out of habit even when we're not really hungry. Along with the very compelling biological signals, these habits can sabotage our efforts at reform.

However, we can also use the same principle to build and strengthen more adaptive food-related behaviors. Part of the strategy involves instituting substitute behaviors that are not compatible with the conditioned, impulsive, "gobble down" habits. For example, substitute behaviors such as: drink lots of water before eating, take a walk when the desire to eat becomes strong, choose healthier, low-density, low-calorie foods instead of or prior to eating previous favorite foods to interrupt the conditioned habit of overeating or eating dense, fatty foods. As these substitute behaviors are integrated and repeated, the conditioning patterns linking the antecedents (hunger and impulse) and consequences (eating healthier foods) also change.

Shape Adaptive Behaviors

Tips to deliberately use reinforcement in our favor to build adaptive behaviors by establishing contingencies between our actions and the "payoff" consequences that follow can *shape* our adaptive eating and food behaviors include:

- Leave the area where you eat immediately after eating. This means *get out of the kitchen or dining area.* Clean up, put food away, then *exit.* The longer you hang around where food is, the more likely your brain will respond to cues to eat more. I discovered that if I go into my bedroom after eating, a remarkable thing happens: ten or fifteen minutes later, I sense my fullness (satiety) and am no longer thinking about extra food or dessert! A simple change of venue changes my mind and appetite. The reinforcement here is the satisfaction that I have eaten enough.

- Include at least one food from the "good/healthy" list (whatever you determine that to be) every day. Eventually, this becomes more automatic as habits build; to start, deliberately introduce (substitute or add) one healthy food that you have typically not eaten regularly in the recent past. Reward yourself from the list of nonedible "payoffs" you determine beforehand.

- Conversely, reward yourself for each day you abstain from "bad" foods. Didn't have dessert or fries today? Good for you! Reinforce the abstention.

- Drink water about twenty minutes before eating to fill your stomach and moderate your appetite. Reward yourself for drinking eight ounces and add more reward for drinking sixteen ounces.

- Practice pushing the plate of food away from you after eating only half to two-thirds of the serving. Serve food on smaller plates. Prepare each meal with reasonable portions.

- Take pictures of everything you eat before starting to eat. At the end of the day, you can see what and how much you ate. As an added benefit toward self-control, document in a log all you ate that day. No need to count calories. Simply observe and record to modify behaviors. This is *self-monitoring*.

- Try intermittent fasting. Be very conservative at first. I recommend skipping dinner once every two weeks to start. This will likely mean that you eat well (and more) earlier in the day, so your blood sugar will maintain at an even level and you won't be tempted to gorge at night. When I go to sleep on a relatively empty stomach, I awaken feeling much better, and my hunger is usually not there until later. A remarkable reset!

- Reward/reinforce yourself for consistently *moving*, and increase your movement gradually. Each person's physical status and capacity is individual. If you are not be able to run, do intense or prolonged exercise, or perhaps even walk much, some type of consistent movement reaps immense benefits—in metabolism, mood, appetite awareness and control, energy and mental focus, and blood flow.

I use and suggest a 10 percent guideline: from baseline, increase your movement by 10 percent each week. If you can walk ten blocks, try walking eleven the next week. Twenty barbell weight repetitions? Try twenty-four the next week. You don't have to keep increasing endlessly; but you'll be surprised at the shaping (behavioral as well as muscular) effect as you increase over a few months.

Important Points About Reinforcement

Consequences that are rewarding or deliver some payoff serve to reinforce our behaviors. Reinforcement happens when behaviors become strengthened or are more likely to reoccur. If you receive a reward without the behavior increasing, then it's not reinforcement—it's just a reward. The overlap between reward and reinforcement always depends upon, and is reflected by, the increase or strengthening of a behavior.

Conversely, behaviors can be reinforced by consequences that are not rewarding or favorable. Yelling or nagging are good examples of reinforcers that are unpleasant but strengthen behaviors. When you yell or nag, you are reinforcing the need to do so in order to get someone to respond to your request, if that gets them to comply. Bad habits such as nail-biting are also reinforced by repetition, though most people would not consider such actions to be rewarding.

To determine whether a behavior is reinforced (regardless of whether or not you want that behavior) you must evaluate the result. If the behavior strengthens or occurs more frequently, then it has been reinforced. As you implement new behaviors around your eating patterns, you will find which consequences are desirable and strong enough to influence your desired outcome. If the promise of buying something you want enables you to constructively and consistently implement some of the changes described above, then you have found a successful contingency to build adaptive behaviors in your eating repertoire.

How to Reduce Unwanted Behaviors

Getting rid of unwanted behaviors is among the most difficult of tasks.[14] It's much easier to shape, increase, and strengthen behaviors into habits than it is to reduce or eliminate them. Reinforcement increases the likelihood that

---

14. For more about the science and practice of modifying behaviors, see extensive descriptions in my book, *Living Intact: Challenge and Choice in Tough Times.*

a behavior will reoccur. Notice how probability is instrumentally threaded throughout nature!

The problem with reducing behaviors intentionally (assuming they are unwanted) is that whenever we pay any attention to a behavior (even just noticing or acknowledging it), we reinforce that behavior (albeit inadvertently). The kicker is that unwanted or nuisance behaviors elicit our attention despite our strongest efforts to ignore them. It's a catch-22. Hunger or cues that signal the appeal of food are very difficult to squelch. We need shaping behaviors that are compatible with the desired ones, and we must also counter the insistence of previously reinforced maladaptive behaviors.

A practical way out of this trap is easy and almost always works. Remember that the *secret to reducing unwanted behaviors is to stop reinforcing them*. Because this is so hard to do, you need a viable alternative that allows you to reinforce what you want, instead of what the other drive (or the environment) manipulates you into reinforcing. Try these:

Shape incompatible responses

Let's say you want to cut down on drinking, smoking, or eating certain foods. First take stock of your patterns by *writing down* the specific dates and actions of your baseline behaviors. Perhaps you are drinking alcohol or eating dessert every day. The probability of indulging daily is 100 percent, ergo the probability of abstinence is zero. Then experiment and ask yourself what is the length of time for which your probability of abstinence is 80 percent? If you drink or eat sweets at 7:00 p.m., then maybe the 80 percent threshold is at 6:00 p.m.. If so, plan two things to happen at 6:00 p.m.:

1. Create a diversion away from drinks and/or sweets. Perhaps plan a larger meal earlier, so you'll be less tempted to indulge subsequently; or plan to be around people or situations where drinks or desserts are not available.

2. Plan and give yourself a substantial nonedible reward to reinforce the likelihood that you will do it again—go one evening without indulging. To be successful when you are trying to turn the tide on an unwanted habit that has the strength and sway

of reinforcement history, you must use the lure of a strong incentive to overcome the power of previously reinforced habits. Substitution and incompatibility of behaviors are key concepts to move you forward in a positive direction.

When you are able to go one day without indulging, rejoice, congratulate yourself (perhaps even tell a confidant), and *make sure to reward yourself with something other than more indulgence in the problem substance*. When ready (probably sooner than you might imagine), try stretching abstinence to two days. Remember to reinforce yourself with the payoff! Eventually, reduced indulgence or abstinence will become a powerful payoff; but in the beginning and interim, use a concrete reward that you will anticipate and enjoy—perhaps something you buy for yourself. Don't worry that you're "bribing" yourself or forming a new overindulgent habit. This strategic tool is used *temporarily* to break a bad habit; you're not likely to become" addicted" to the intervening tool. You will become accustomed to the new and more positive habit. When this happens, the need to keep reinforcing it materially will fade.

Use response costs to reduce unwanted behaviors

A *response cost* is a consequence that predictably follows a behavior, one that costs the person exhibiting an undesirable or against-the-rules behavior. For example, a parking ticket is a response cost, something you must pay for committing an infraction. Response costs are effective tools for reducing unwanted behaviors, because they are predictable expectations or impositions of penalties. Imposing a cost upon the bad behavior has a deterrent effect instead of a reinforcing effect you may not intend (such as when you yell, threaten, or criticize the behavior).

- Response costs involve very little work on your part, once *you* set up the rules and contingencies (if you do this, then you pay that).
- Response costs are very economical, since they don't add rewards.
- Response costs can be material (such as forfeiting money or possessions for a period of time)—or they can be costs imposed

in the form of *work*, e.g., if you overindulge, you can link that to paying a consequence such as promptly doing some extra chores (housework, unpleasant or odious activities like cleaning the toilet, etc.). I do not advise using exercise as a response cost to poor eating because this tends to backfire and lead to self-punishment and reduced motivation.

- Response costs can include temporarily restricting preferred activities: e.g., "Since I ate that unhealthy food today, I will deliberately not watch TV or use my computer recreationally this evening." Other potential response costs:
  - Forfeit devices for a short, specified time period.
  - Pay extra money to a family member or charity.
  - Do menial, repetitive work (such as cleaning, writing apologies, organizing files; even busy work like transferring 200 pennies from one jar to another).
  - Record and/or deliver verbal apologies to family members.
- Response costs can include temporarily restricting preferred activities. Since response costs are very effective ways to introduce a predictable association between undesirable behaviors (typically with a conditioned high probability) and a consequence—payment—that has a deterrent effect with an eventual reduction in the behavior due to the cost of indulging in it, response costs are not punishment. Whereas punishment involves a significantly adverse consequence (sometimes painful) that has the effect of reducing or suppressing a behavior, a response cost is a cost—not intended to be hurtful, but to instill by association the knowledge that indulging in certain behaviors is expensive. That is the deterring effect.

Probability

Whether we want to change, predict, or interpret behaviors and events, we use probability to inform expectations and responses to what might or will occur. Probability indicates the *likelihood* of something *occurring or reoccurring*.

Consciously or otherwise, we use probability principles constantly to interpret, plan, prepare, and modify our understanding and responses internally and to our world. The behavioral rules governing reinforcement and habits described above are underpinned and influenced by probability. You can use these probability principles strategically to aid your adoption of better eating habits. A review of how probability operates in daily life will help you utilize its power to control your eating and weight.

Probability examples in everyday life

We typically think of probability as a mathematician's formulaic assessment of how likely it is that an event will occur—and that's true. However, we use probability all the time to predict what's likely to happen in everyday life and to assess the risks and benefits of particular courses of action.

You use probability every time you change lanes on a highway. Prior to your move to change lanes, you calculate the risk that another vehicle will be in your way and potentially result in a collision. This is so automatic and routine that you hardly think of changing lanes as a risk assessment; but it is, even though you don't consciously use a math formula. In less familiar traffic or weather conditions, you may pay more attention to your decision-making and adjust your driving accordingly. When making driving decisions, you "win" at such a high percentage of the time (you don't get into accidents), that the probability algorithms you subconsciously and routinely use happen "under the radar" of your conscious planning.

Industries such as banking and insurance would not be profitable if they didn't rely on probability data to make astute business decisions about lending and rates. Athletes and coaches use probability to anticipate their opponents' tactical moves and strategies and to adjust their own performance and defenses. Good test-takers anticipate what questions and topics will be covered on the exams. Keen businesspeople handle presentations and customer interactions by preparing for likely concerns and objections. Government agencies use probability to assess the threat and risk of terrorism. Doctors, scientists, and researchers use statistics to predict the likelihood of developing a disease, acquiring an infection, or healing from an injury. Dating services and law enforcement utilize probability to profile behavior. Planning committees use probability to predict future growth and community needs.

We all use probability daily in a myriad of ways from guiding ordinary functioning to predicting the most likely outcomes in novel or unfamiliar situations. We combine past experience with current conditions to anticipate how soon we will really need to use a bathroom or how long we can go without eating before becoming fatigued or irritable. We rely on probability to forecast people's reactions to our emotions, overtures, and grievances. We form preferences, biases, and even prejudices based on our accumulated personal data with people and situations bearing similarities to what we previously experienced.

Given our inherent and integral need to assess risk, predict outcomes, and modify our actions and expectations, it's not surprising that the awareness and facile manipulation of probabilities plays a key role in success in so many areas of life. You don't need complicated formulas or computer-assisted statistical models. You only need to develop and hone your skills of observation and analysis, drawing upon the accumulation of your experiences. From these experiences, you make *assessments of cause and effect,* you refine your ability to *recognize and compare categories* of experience (past and present), and you astutely sift from your experiences the *essential similarities, differences, and essential organizing principles* that will allow you to more accurately interpret the likely outcomes of your choices and behaviors interacting with the circumstances and challenges you face.

You can use probability to improve your chances of eating better and becoming healthier.

Example 1: Self-discipline and routine

Certain "tricks" reliably help me avoid overeating and eating sweets. These propensities combine probability with frequency and duration to keep me satisfied and sustainable on a dietary regimen I've determined is better for me.

I've made these observations reliably over time about how my own behaviors with food influence my desired and logistical outcomes. Since I sleep better and feel better the next morning when I go to bed on less than a full stomach, and I know that the more sweets and carbs I eat, the more I tend to want. So I take advantage of certain techniques to tilt the odds in my favor. If I eat moderate amounts of quality protein and fat before my blood sugar dips, I become satisfied with small portions and few or no carbs. If I eat less and eat earlier in the evening, I rest and feel better. If I avoid sweets, my desire for them dwindles in proportion to how much and how often I eat them.

These observations are also intertwined with frequency, duration, and probability. The less frequently I stuff myself or eat unhealthy foods, the less I *want* them. A definite scientific nutritional relationship is a work here; but in this example, I'm emphasizing the *correlative observation*. It may seem counterintuitive, but I feel less deprived the less often and the longer I go without indulging myself.

As I indulge less frequently, the probability that I will indulge decreases (a good thing). To boot, the longer I go without indulging or eating in excess, the more likely this habit will establish itself as the new normal, and the easier it is for me to continue on a healthy pattern. I've found that eating ice cream (because I "deserve" it) just leads to wanting more ice cream the next day. Consider that, once in a while, ice cream is okay. But for me, *thinking about it* requires too much stress and work. I need my physiology to cooperate to make life easier. I have lots of ice cream in my freezer in multiple favorite flavors. I eat ice cream once every few months or less frequently. I love ice cream, but it's a wicked tempter, and the habit of abstinence simply works better for me.

Once I exit from the kitchen or family room (where I usually relax after dinner) and go to my bedroom, my desire for dessert drops dramatically. How uncanny that I can think about and crave dessert in one room, but moving thirty steps away, after brushing my teeth, eradicates my desire for any more food, including carbs! Funny coincidence, but I capitalize on it.

Additionally, I noticed that eating a handful of grapes or berries satisfies my sweet tooth and eliminates the craving for processed or high-sugar foods. Though the nutritional underpinning for that effect is solid, the message here is that we can positively change the probabilities surrounding our eating behaviors by strategic observations and cause-and-effect interventions.

Example 2: Movement and exercise

Probabilities are similarly influential and modifiable concerning my exercise routines. The more hours that elapse during the day, the less likely I am to exercise. Even if I have more time later in the day, I am less likely to exercise. So if I'm going to work out, I better do it early in the day. Therefore, I follow the habit and plan and execute my gym visits earlier. This leads to more frequency, greater intensity, and longer duration of exercise. After I exercise, I almost always feel much better! This spirals into a habit of higher probability that I will exercise regularly.

Observation and habit are great companions to reinforce the company of success and confidence if you treat them with respect and garner their wisdom.

Example 3: Stretch periods of abstinence

As we all know, breaking habits can be quite difficult. Even when the outcomes of our habits are destructive or dire, the power of reinforcement can keep us stuck doing what we don't ultimately want to do.

Since we tend to keep doing what we've done before, we can use the principles of shaping (small steps of change), reinforcement, and probability to gradually modify our eating behaviors. The key is to progressively lengthen the time periods between indulgences in the undesired behaviors. As an example, say you want to forgo sweet desserts. With effort and perhaps "white-knuckling" resistance, you manage to cut down your frequency of indulgence. But you still revert to temptation and eat those sweets regularly. The goal would be to gradually increase the number of days you go *without* eating those foods.

a. Assess a baseline for several time periods in which the behavior occurs regularly. At this starting point use the data from this baseline assessment that you have dessert six days per week. A starting goal might be to go a day or two without dessert.

b. If you do go a day without dessert, provide yourself with a reward/reinforcement *right away*. It's vital to deliver the payoff promptly so the new behavior is associated directly with the payoff.

c. Observe how many days you can go without dessert. Don't berate yourself for backsliding or relapse—you are strategically working on new habits. Let's say that over two weeks, you can comfortably achieve two days at a time before you give in—fine. Even if that becomes your new pattern, you are abstaining from dessert two more days than previously. Just don't stop there.

d. Try to stretch your abstinence to three consecutive days. Reward yourself heavily at the beginning to get a new habit off the ground. You can fade back and thin the rewards after you are more consistently successful. The new habit will continue through intermittent reinforcement with less-frequent payoffs. By observing your behavior, your temptations, and your obsessive preoccupations with desiring foods on the "bad' list, assign a probability value in terms of percentages to short periods of time corresponding to "good behavior" (absence of transgressions). For example, the probability you can go one day without dessert may be 90 percent; but the probability you can go two days may be 80 percent; and the probability that you can go a week is 10 percent. As you can see (or graph), as time without or between transgressions increases, the probability of continued good behavior decreases. Thus you have a predictability model using probabilities estimated from your observations.

e. Schedule a positive reinforcement somewhere around the 80 percent probability that abstinence continues. That is, deliberately intervene and reward the "good behavior," which is the absence of indulgence or relapse. Using this example above, you would reward yourself sometime before the end of the second day of no dessert. The reason for this is that people tend to learn most effectively at a reinforcement rate somewhere around 80 percent. Above that success rate, the person feels good, but little new learning or improvements occur. As the reinforcement probability drops significantly, the challenge becomes too great, discouragement ensues, and motivation and effort decrease.

f. As you can go more intervals without dessert—say over a month you skip dessert two days each week—try skipping dessert at least three consecutive days. When you are successful at this, a remarkably helpful change occurs: not only do you save calories and feel better about yourself: along with this *your brain and body become acclimated to loner periods of no dessert*. This new pattern becomes the norm!

g. Pretty soon you'll be able to stretch the abstinence to weeks (eventually longer) without eating or depending upon dessert. Using this gradual shaping method, your biological and behavioral systems will establish no desert as the new normal. Eating dessert will become the aberration. *Voila*—a new adaptive habit takes shape!

h. You can use this method for abstaining from other indulgences— foods, alcohol, smoking, drugs, etc.

The power of probability is forceful and awesome. Practice harnessing it in your favor to take charge and gain better control over your eating and relationship with food.

Probability can lull you into bad habits. By learning and using its predictability models and strategically implementing reinforcement, you improve your chances of achieving winning outcomes.

Remember these wise words: if you keep doing more of what you're doing, you'll likely get more of what you've got, and the classic definition of insanity is doing the same thing again and again but expecting different results.

CHAPTER 13

What to Eat

I will not tell anyone else what to eat. I will only advise from my own knowledge and experience of what works for me, along with a brief distillation of common medical and nutritional information and best practices concerning food and metabolism. In a book about weight loss, you might expect reliable specifics about foods that shed pounds. However, such advice is not always applicable or advisable to a wide range of individuals, even though the basic principles make sense. Individual bodies work differently—common biological principles notwithstanding, and people have a wide range of preferences and tolerances for dietary regimens. So I have no rigid formulas for do's and don'ts to recommend. Instead, I share what has worked for me and what I discovered that help to relieve my temptations and hunger, and avoid my deprivation and suffering.

My Transition

My diet and eating habits changed gradually over the years. For the decades when I was heavy, I ordered or prepared large amounts of food. The habit of eating way too much calorie-dense food made me full after first eating, but I soon needed to eat more as my blood sugar rebounded uncomfortably. The foods I ate were salty, fatty, and loaded with sweeteners and additives that produced cravings for more of the same.

I tried many different dietary programs: gluten-free diets, ketogenic fare, fat-free regimens, etc. Some induced weight loss, but none of it lasted. Those diets became boring, restrictive, and unsustainable. This may sound familiar to you.

In 2018, I had quadruple bypass open heart surgery, something I would not care to repeat. That saved my life and notified me that it was time to make significant life changes, particularly in my diet. For most of my life, I had been a voracious carnivore. For me, vegetables (most of which I always liked) were a capitulation to justify my mainstay of rich and fatty animal foods. Like the vast majority of Americans, I had a staple diet of cows, pigs, and chickens as my main courses. Tasty indeed, but I decided this was no longer for me. I decided to give up eating meat.

My decision was partly ethical, but mostly based on the very convincing evidence from the scientific research and books I read. The most compelling among these was *China Study: The Most Comprehensive Study of Nutrition Ever Conducted* by T. Colin Campbell, PhD, and Thomas M. Campbell, MD. This book chronicles meticulous longitudinal studies documenting the very real relationship between eating meat and many diseases.

My Diet

Let me emphasize that my change of diet has been gradual (and still evolving). This has been partly intentional and partly the result of the way that eating differently affected my taste preferences, gut feelings (literally), appetite and gastro modulation (self-regulation), and satiety with different foods. As I relinquished eating processed meats, such as sausages, hot dogs, salami, etc., then other red meats (the burgers and steaks I used to love), and then chicken, I noticed a steady reduction in my blood pressure and cholesterol, and my desire for sweets lessened. Since animal foods, particularly flesh, contain a lot of salt, I also found a reduction in thirst and bloating after heavier meals. Meat takes longer to digest than many foods, and my system felt clearer and cleaner without it.

Good sources of protein are necessary. Without animal foods, it was important to be mindful and consistent in consuming good quality protein. Plant foods contain protein, but not necessarily in the amounts supplied by similar quantities of animal foods. I still eat fish a few times per week. In moderate amounts, fish provides excellent protein and healthier fat than meat. I eat eggs and egg products intermittently, usually about once or twice a week.

I cut way back on dairy products—no milk for decades, ice cream indulgences (a weakness for me) maybe twice a year, occasional yogurt or sour cream. I used to eat fresh fruit with yogurt or cream, but gradually transitioned to do without it. In my indulgent days, I embellished rich ice cream or gelato with a bath of heavy cream: delicious, but too much! This was the biggest problem for me: whenever I ate ice cream, I craved it again the next day. I had to fight the craving and ended up playing mind games with myself about strategic schedules to satisfy and cater to what I thought I "deserved." This merry-go-round, and having to limit my portions, turned out to be way-too-much *work*. It was easier to just stay away from ice cream. I still find it delicious, but I no longer miss it.

I love cheeses, but they contain a lot of salt and saturated fat. I occasionally have a grilled cheese sandwich, a cheesy omelet, or eggplant parmesan. And I eat pizza. But, whereas I used to eat pizza two or three times a week, I now indulge about every two weeks. I eat one or two slices instead of my previous habit of three or four at a time.

I eat dried, grated cheeses: Parmesan and Romano sprinkled on pasta. My main "sellout" indulgence is butter. I love bread and butter. I would rather have whole grain bread with butter than most other foods. A slice (or two if I've exercised a lot) is deeply satisfying. I seem to get away with it—though, in general, breads are not a good staple for health or weight control. My moderate bread habit substitutes satisfactorily for other processed carbohydrates. However, I love pasta! I eat small to moderate amounts of pasta once or twice a week (with butter or olive oil, grated cheese, and lots of pepper).

In keeping with my reduced appetite, I usually have two servings of fresh vegetables (cooked or raw) along with fish, or pasta, or bread.

The Jewish boy in me will very occasionally indulge in a *shmear* (cream cheese) on a bagel with lox and green onions. However, this is now a heavy meal for me; so I usually eat only half of one such sandwich.

Transformational Substitution

Several years ago, I discovered a plant-based, nutrition shake that has become a daily staple for me. Many such shake varieties on the market contain natural organic superfoods and essential nutrients in an all-in-one meal. The one I use now is called Ka'Chava. Almost every morning, I blend a rich-tasting shake from two capfuls of Ka'Chava along with ice and a banana. The shake is delicious, filling, and satisfying! Including the banana, it is less than 400 calories. This usually allays my hunger and sits comfortably in my gut, allowing me to move around or even exercise without heaviness, which was never the case in my former days of breakfasts of bacon, eggs, refined toast, and sometimes pancakes. The plant-based "superfood" is clean, light, nutritious, and low in calories. If I am hungry in the afternoon, I may have some dried fruit or vegetable chip snack. I get through the day with gut satisfaction, energy, and a calorie deficit that allows for a richer dinner.

Foods I Eat

I hope my own experiences and personal disclosures here will be helpful.

- Fresh vegetables I eat daily include leafy greens (lots of kale, spinach, and bok choy); carrots, parsnips, beets; squash; lots of onions (red, green, and white).

- Tofu is a staple ingredient that is low-calorie, light but filling, and absorbs and blends with tastes of many foods. I am partial to Asian foods, which use tofu in many classic dishes, Indian curries, Korean and Japanese dishes and soups, and many varieties of Chinese cooking. I eat something with tofu almost every day.

- Chick peas have become my new romance! Blended in salads with beans and onions, mashed and flavored with spices and oil in traditional hummus, cooked into crunchy falafel. Filling, satisfying, versatile, low-calorie, and very nutritious—chick peas have become a main go-to food for weight control and healthy, moderate eating.

128

- Beans are a staple. I eat all kinds and try to rotate a variety. I like pinto beans and black beans. I often buy them cooked from Mexican eateries (not refried beans, which have pork fat), such as kidney beans, favas, and for a treat, baked beans (though they are sweetened).

- Pickled vegetables. I have become enamored with various pickled vegetable preparations. I'm particularly fond of a traditional Korean dish called kimchi. Though salty, it is full of fiber, extremely vibrant and tasty (particularly if you like hot, spicy foods), low-calorie, and satisfying. Pickled vegetables are full of nutrients, including probiotics and antioxidants. A few forkfuls deliver satisfying taste and a slight onset of sweat that reduces appetite.

- Lentils are healthy nutritionally and have been shown to reduce blood pressure and cholesterol. They are full of fiber and are great for the gut biome. However I admit that I still force myself to include lentils regularly. To me, they are not that tasty, though they are easily adapted to flavorful recipes in many traditional cultures. Lentils and chickpeas are among the healthiest foods one can eat.

- Salads are a necessary staple: filling, healthy, delicious in many varieties and iterations. Raw food is the best. In colder weather, salads tend to be less satisfying, but I include them anyway.

- Soups are a dieter's godsend. The liquid base of soups make them ideal for blended tastes, hearty cooked satisfaction, and inclusion and absorption of many different food sources. I have to admit, I can be easily seduced by creamy soups and bisques. I give in once in a while.

- Fish. I love many kinds. I eat salmon once or twice a week. I also eat cod, tuna, halibut, sole, yellowtail, swordfish, and others on an intermittent rotating basis. I eat clams intermittently. I enjoy shrimp in moderation and occasional indulgence in crab, lobster, or oysters, or calamari. I avoid frozen fish, as fresh fish is superior in flavor. One must be careful in the purchase, transportation, and storage, and cook fresh fish soon after purchase. Good fresh fish is expensive, so it is an indulgence and a luxury for many. I am fortunate to be able to include it in my diet. Fish supplies great protein with low-to-moderate amounts of fat and omegas. Two to four ounces of fish is light, satisfying, protein rich, and low in fat.

- Eggs. Once a week or so, I make plain poached or fried eggs. Every few weeks I have an omelet, plain or with grated cheese and/or spinach. Eggs are often included as emulsifiers in dressings and baked goods. Occasionally I have Mexican chili rellenos (without meat).

- Pasta. I am a sucker for pasta. I can't seem to give it up. I eat far less in one sitting than I used to, but I need my pasta fix, usually rigatoni, fettuccini, or fusilli, with olive oil and/or butter and some grated cheese and pepper. I also like Asian pasta dishes such as lo mein or chow fun with vegetables. I have a deal with myself whereby I must *earn* these carbs. That means plentiful exercise and limitations on other calorie-dense foods on the days I eat pasta. Though whole-grain, unrefined pastas are much healthier, I don't like the taste. I go with the refined pastas and discipline myself in other food choices.

- Rice is not my favorite, although I do occasionally enjoy fried rice with fresh vegetables or kimchi.

- Bread is my necessary weakness: bread and butter—so satisfying that I believe it enables me to stay on the wagon with most of my other food limitations. The occasional white refined bagel or crunchy roll satisfies that spongy, pillowy mouth feel. I allow myself that indulgence once in a while. Usually, I buy freshly baked, whole grain sourdough at a local bakery. One or two slices, three or four times a week is enough to spoil me with a feast.

- Desserts. I rarely eat cakes, muffins, etc. When I do, I prefer the less-sweet confections such as bread pudding. No cookies, and ice cream very rarely. Once or twice a week, I'll eat fresh fruit in season—a pear, a peach, an apple. Sometimes, to cap off my dinner, I'll have three tablespoons of unsweetened apple sauce.

- Chips. I'm allergic to potatoes (odd, I know), so I do not eat potato products (chips, fries, etc.). I have a fondness for corn chips. I occasionally indulge in homemade vegetarian nachos, sprinkled with cheese and flavored with soy sauce. I use low-fat salsas for enhancement. When I eat out (and very hungry waiting for the meal), I allow myself to snack on corn chips and guacamole. As my diet has evolved, I find that chips and cheese become too heavy. I indulge in these foods less and less. Crackers are addictive poisons I eschew (not chew).

- Nuts are nutritious (especially without oils or natural from the shells), better than chips, but still high in fat and calories. If you can eat a small handful in place of chips, you may feel satisfied and be better off. I can't do that. I want to eat the whole can. So I rarely eat nuts, except when they are used to adorn cooked dishes or salads.

- Snacks. I snack on dried fruits most days, usually two to four dried prunes, apricots, or apples. Once or twice a week, I eat fresh fruit in season—a pear, peach, or apple. I keep a variety of low-fat, unsweetened fruit and vegetable chips in my pantry and car. Several times a day (especially after a gym workout or when driving home after work) I will eat several handfuls of vegetable chips or dried apple chips. A variety of tasty, satisfying dried vegetable chips of all kinds are available—such as cauliflower, beet, carrot, lily pops, etc. I read labels and avoid fats and sweeteners. The ones I eat generally have about 120 calories per portion; half a portion satisfies me. But be careful. So many of these products with creative and alluring names are fat and calorie dense. A four-ounce bag can stuff you with a thousand calories from bad fats and sweeteners of different names. Beware of fats, sugars, and too much salt, surreptitiously saturated into many "health foods." Go for the ones flavored with cheese or seaweed powder, sea salt, or other spices. Many varieties of these products are available online. They keep well without preservatives. Some of my favorites are naked beet chips, cauliflower tubes, and popped lily seeds.

- Beverages. I drink only tap water, sparkling water, and black coffee. I'm satisfied with those and need nothing else. No alcohol, soft drinks, juices, milk or fruit shakes, none of it. They offer too many calories, rebounding blood sugar highs and lows and addiction. I'm not suggesting that you restrict yourself to what I drink (which doesn't feel like restriction whatsoever to me). I'm simply reporting what I've become quite satisfied with in fluids over time (decades actually).

- Food preparation. I used to cook quite a bit, and I enjoyed entertaining. Those habits have diminished as I grow older, eat out far less often, and turn my attention to more focused and selective activities. I spend limited time at the stove, usually preferring to heat and reheat food in the oven. I buy prepared foods from restaurants and ethnic shops, spending extra on food I know is prepared with fresh ingredients from scratch. I am fortunate to afford this, and I realize that many are on limited budgets and by necessity must prepare and cook at home. Carried out with good information, patience, and prudence, this necessity carries a silver lining in that you know and control what goes into your meals and your stomach.

I cook fish and vegetables, casseroles, and pastas. I use high-quality vegetable oils (olive, sunflower, sesame), and I sauté, bake, and broil. I love deep-fried foods, yet never prepare those at home (too dangerous for me). I will occasionally buy onion rings or fried fish from markets or restaurants. However, I find that my reaction to fried foods is more sensitive than it used to be. Whereas I used to eat a whole bag of onion rings, now I occasionally eat one to three, quickly reaching my saturation with greasy food. I no longer have a need for the large portions I took for granted as necessary for so much of my gustatory life. And I am happier and healthier and grateful for those changes.

Many health-conscious circles emphasize the importance of organic foods. Where possible, choosing organic foods limits the additives and preservatives that otherwise may saturate produce and manufactured foods. Organic foods are typically more expensive. An added benefit from organic produce is the reduction of farmworker exposure to pesticides that are not good for workers—or for our gut.

In sum, I enjoy a wide variety of foods that nourish, satisfy, and sustain me. I have managed to lose a lot of weight and keep it off without feeling deprived or suffering, or missing out or feeling hungry too often, or becoming overly obsessed with negative thoughts or behaviors over food. I've gradually adapted to a healthier diet, one that keeps my blood sugar even and controlled and a pattern of eating that is satisfying, sustainable, and good for my body and mind.

You can do this too. But you must determine what works for *you*—some of it through reading, some with good medical advice, and some through personal preferences seasoned with trial-and-error experimentation.

CHAPTER 14

Downsize

As we form an identity and seek our place in the world, efforts to acquire, achieve, and gain (*get*) abound. This is part and parcel of finding a stake in life, a sense of belonging, security, and a set of preferences and beliefs. When we are younger, opportunities may invite, and appetites and energy are usually strong. As we explore the goodies and sample the bounty, we feed tastes and build habits of indulgence according to availability and affordability.

With age, metabolism slows, physical prowess eventually declines, and most of us become more sedentary. Nevertheless we tend to eat the same or more, despite an inevitable reduced need for calories. To boot, with advancing age, our bodies have less tolerance for rich foods and alcohol, even in the absence of encroaching or acquired medical problems.

Eventually it's time to downsize. Empty nesters or retirees may consider the need for less house and fewer possessions. Financial hardship may prompt a downsizing lifestyle due to necessity. And of course, the pervasive problem of weight gain saddles and afflicts a majority. The time has come to downsize the body—a difficult but doable endeavor.

A Desirable Club

Bodybuilders and 98-pound weaklings who get sand kicked at them on the beach strive to get bigger. The rest of us usually want to get smaller. Among those fortunate to succeed at weight loss, a milestone with a peculiar name is the *Onederful Club*. The name refers to getting body weight under 200 pounds, an enviable achievement for the minions who struggle with diet and obesity. A person of any weight may want to lose some pounds, and this may be desirable, helpful, appropriate, vain, etc. For a competitive athlete, a model, an entertainment star, and others, losing a few pounds can make a difference in health, appearance, and confidence.

The reality is that most people who are "fat" exceed 200 pounds, many by scores above that. Except for very tall people, or outliers, the human frame and organs are not built to support weights exceeding 200 pounds, and certainly not by a lot. Therefore, weight-loss progress that dips below the significant number is a glorious milestone and often a harbinger of further weight reduction.

Ducking under 200 pounds may not be the finish line, but it's a mile marker that attests to persistence and success. You won't see these people wearing labels, and they don't give out symbols as in AA or other twelve-step programs. But those in the Onederful Club are proud and confident, and it's noticeable in their appearance.

Weight-Loss Benefits

The obvious benefits to losing weight include:

- Better health
- More energy
- Improved appearance
- More confidence
- Better clothing fit
- Possible new clothing and styles
- Easier movement
- Less wear and tear on joints
- Praise and notice from others
- Healing of ailments and sometimes medical conditions (e.g., diabetes, high blood pressure
- Less medication
- Better sleep

- Motivation for old and new activities
- Eligibility for surgeries where obesity may incur risks and complications

If weight loss is achieved gradually, safely, and appropriately, a newer and less-obsessive relationship with food and eating can also evolve. Such downsizing brings many compounded benefits.

Downsize Surprises

Other surprising benefits accrue with weight loss, some pleasant and some odd. Typical Americans have increased significantly in body size over the past half-century. Although commercial interests have gradually adapted the sizes and manufacturing patterns of consumer products, overweight people generally struggle with fitting (comfortably or at all) into seats in theaters, on airplanes, and even cars. To find that you can fit into clothing and commercial furniture comfortably and with room to spare is a delightful surprise.

I am reminded of a story that sardonically illustrates the point:

With great effort and persistence, a chronically obese woman managed to lose 150 pounds. At her heaviest, she could barely move without pain and rarely left the house. Thrilled with her new body, she was proudly able to attend her daughter's school play. She wiggled into the elementary school auditorium seat, a feat that was previously unthinkable. Yet she was still a large person.

As the play began, a man sitting behind her tapped her on the shoulder and said, "Lady, you're blocking my view. Why don't you lose some weight?"

Some people are inveterately mean.

Nonetheless, what an achievement it is to fit in and be more fit!

Odd surprises

I enjoy clothing and have a prolific wardrobe. Over the years, I've spent a lot of money accumulating closets full of clothes in many sizes (mostly extra-large).

As my weight loss progressed, my clothes became loose and eventually baggy. This development was a great boon to my tailor, who profited immensely from my repeated patronization. (What a blessing!) Although I bought new clothes, I wanted to keep my collection of expensive and still-stylish garb. Before tailoring, many of my pants needed to be cinched at the waist by a tightened belt. Still, the cut of the fabric was originally sewn in a much larger size. Therefore, even with cinching and eventual tailoring, the pockets rotated to odd and unflattering positions on my body—with some, the side pockets shifted almost to the rear!

As my pants fit looser, I found that my wallet and phone fell out with regularity. I needed to be more vigilant to not lose things. In former days, I needed to unbutton my trousers after a meal—quite the hidden embarrassment in restaurants.

I am short in stature. Almost every garment I purchase needs to be shortened in sleeves and pant length. I take this for granted. But with substantial weight loss, even the shirt sleeves that were originally shortened needed to be shortened further by a cuff length due to the reduced body size. Amazing!

I have long given up eating at buffets. Who needs that?! I am no longer an "endurance" eater trying to beat the system by overindulgence in all-you-can-eat. I still get hungry daily, and I really enjoy eating, but now I fill up quickly. So I spend less money on quantity and more on quality and fresh food. No bargains, no supersize, no *Your order comes with* (these extra calories).

As mentioned earlier, one of the most intriguing surprises on my weight-loss journey has been the evolution and transition in my taste and food preferences. After a lifetime of savoring and seeking rich, fatty, and fried foods, I find that I rarely crave them now. I have become accustomed to lighter, less dense, less processed food. When I eat rich foods, I feel "heavier" physically, a less comfortable state than when I eat lighter. And it comes naturally—no struggle or deprivation. If I eat onion rings or pizza, I have a small portion, not out of discipline, but because a little is plenty. More is not better or more satisfying. For me, this has been a truly remarkable transformation.

Environmental and Social Ripples

For environmentalists or the climate conscious, consider that lighter passengers require less airplane fuel—better for the carbon imprint! Thinner people means more seats that fit in a limited space—more profit for airlines and more comfort for passengers. The apparel industries stand to profit as newly skinny people need newer clothes and fashions. Fitness industries are booming. Gyms, home fitness equipment, personal trainers, and coaches are among the economic profiteers from weight-loss endeavors.

The monolithic food manufacturers are being called to task for their ruthless processing methods that garner huge profits at the population's expense of poor health. This must change, and so it will.

In the healthcare sector, a mainstay of our national economy, treating chronic illness is exorbitantly expensive. We are patching a dam and fleeing from a tsunami—not preserving health or resources. Somehow—and I believe this will begin to happen sooner rather than later—we as a society must transition from treating and rescuing disease (in mostly losing battles) caused by poor diet, to promoting good health by sound nutrition, rational policies, healthcare stipends, and insurance-covered preventive care.

We have better science than ever before. We know more about healthy and varied nutrition and the dietary causes of diseases than in any previous era. We have marvelous and improving technology in the biological (including genetic), pharmaceutical, and behavioral realms. As a society, we (and you as an individual) can program, change, control, and transform the way we eat, think about, and produce food.

Though my ancestry and family history predisposed me to certain health problems, a lot of my genes didn't fit. But I've lost lots of weight as well as many of the habits and beliefs that once weighed and wore me down. In most ways, I am the same person—just thinner, healthier, and more mature.

Life always involves some deprivation and suffering that we must confront, accept, and look beyond. But we also have the power and the tools to stop bearing deprivation and suffering in our obsessions and behaviors with food and with our body; we can achieve vastly improved health and happiness.

CHAPTER 15

Become Friends With Yourself and With Food

As pointed out throughout this book, my intention is not just to help people lose unwanted weight. Just as important, I want all of us to come to better terms with our body image, our feelings about ourselves, and our enjoyment of and relationship with food.

If you are reading this book because you have been frustrated and disappointed in battling weight and eating habits for a long time, it seems implicit that you will feel better and like yourself more if you lose weight, keep it off, and improve and control your eating habits. Not so fast though. While this may be true, for so many the struggle with food, eating, and body image appears ongoing, even if and when *substantial weight loss is achieved*. Many people—fat, thin, and in-between—somehow accept themselves even when they fall short of their goals or they don't adore their bodies, features, or some parts of themselves. Self-acceptance and appropriate confidence and pride in one's characteristics do not correlate neatly with appearance or girth.

While it follows that significant and commendable weight loss typically does result in better confidence and satisfaction, relying upon such as a barometer and arbiter of success and positive self-esteem is laden with pitfalls, owing to the precarious foundations of self-respect and self-image with which most people struggle.

Why Hate Yourself?

A strange and inimical reality is that many people are at war with themselves. Intentionally or incidentally, they expose and deprecate themselves under the harsh, unforgiving lights of self-criticism, unfavorable comparisons, and self-loathing.

Many of these self-critical tendencies are products of years of shaming, ostracism, criticism, and demanding standards from parents along with pressure from society's images and implied expectations: standards of beauty extolled from fashion, movie stars and icons, social media, and the internalized standards of idolatry that people take upon themselves. Though clearly not limited to females, women often bear more of the burden from the pressures and stereotypes that contribute to not feeling or looking good enough. Idealized standards of beauty—particularly feminine beauty—are quite narrow and unrealistic.

Added to the sociocultural and developmental factors that make people deplore themselves and their looks are the negative mind habits that afflict so many with obsessive compulsive thinking and worrying. Those boggled with the torturing internal loops of obsessive and intrusive thoughts often worry about, grapple with, and fear a variety of "what ifs" that decimate peace of mind. In the constellation of repetitive thoughts that beset such individuals, respite might be temporarily achieved through various treatments and exercises. For the person who cringes when looking in the mirror (and keeps thinking about their image negatively), self-infliction is incessant.

Escape From Self

For many who engage in relentless self-criticism and self-loathing, relief is grasped through self-medication. This may include alcohol, drugs, and/or—of course—food.

Along with the neurobiochemical addictions that can develop, a psychological habituation state can occur that is triggered by and tied to overeating. Food coma is an epithet describing the physiological state of torpor and numbing that accrues through binge eating. When the bloodstream is flooded with glucose and the stomach is stuffed, cravings and anxiety give way to *temporary* palliation and preoccupation with digestion.

With practice (dysfunctional and addictive practice), the brain and gut develop associations for fullness that are truly unhealthy physically and psychologically. A stinging joke goes, "My cue to stop eating is when I am flooded with sufficiently hating myself."

Friends

This chapter title, "Becoming Friends With Yourself and Food," is emblematic of my purpose to keep front and center the importance of *feeling good about yourself* regardless of your weight (even as you try to lose and control it). Your weight notwithstanding, it's essential to develop a healthy and comfortable relationship with your identity (which includes your body image) and your relationship with food and how you eat and think about it.

With that in mind, let's look at what friendship means.

What does friendship involve and what is it for?

We can describe friendship as including the following:

- Affinity—having a liking or feeling of attraction for someone;
- Trust—intimate feelings of safety and comfort in confiding, no fear of betrayal;
- Healthy interest—genuine interest in a friend's opinions, needs, and activities;
- Companionship—being and doing things together in fellowship;
- Sharing—exchanging experiences, feelings, and possessions;
- Dependability—reliability, being able to count on one another with confidence;
- Reciprocation—mutual giving and taking; doing things for each other;
- Anticipation—eagerness and looking forward to someone's company or shared experience and communication; and

- Forgiveness—letting go of grudges, resentment, or desire for payback or getting even; overlooking disappointment.

These common aspects of friendship are usually understood in the context of a relationship with another person. But how might these same characteristics apply to one's relationship with oneself? And with our relationship with food and eating?

Liking and feeling good about oneself is a foundation for confidence, acceptance, and reasonable standards in holding expectations for self and others. We must be able to trust ourself, and that is built upon experience, judgment, and discernment. No one makes all the right decisions; but believing in your own ability and judgment allows for better clarity in careful choices.

We need to place value on our own opinions and the legitimacy of our needs and feelings. This goes along with flexibility and a degree of open-mindedness to differing points of view.

Just as we can and should enjoy relating to others, we should develop self-reliance and a level of comfort in being with ourself, notwithstanding that temperaments differ with regard to the desire for socialization versus solitary activities. They are not mutually exclusive. If you are very uncomfortable with your body or place too much stock or sensitivity in your appearance, you will have difficulty disclosing, sharing, or even accepting the views and feelings that others have toward you. Despite the logic and wisdom of being kind to yourself, self-criticism, perfectionistic standards, and even self-flagellation are rampant among those who struggle with weight and body image.

Becoming friends with yourself—mind, body, habits, flaws, and mistakes—requires reasonable standards and goals combined with acceptance and forgiveness, applied inwardly. I suggest no magic formula, only guidelines gradually developed and internalized to become increasingly *okay* with who we are, even as we strive to be better.

Self-acceptance accrues through experience; but it also benefits from the input of trusted advisors, knowledgeable experts, and people who have walked in our life shoes.

Friends With Your Brain and With Food

Becoming friends with your brain may seem like an odd combination or juxtaposition of identity and self-regard. However, it has specific and practical meaning. Knowing yourself over time involves a realistic and evidentiary assessment of your strengths, weaknesses, temptations, blind spots, and—so importantly—the way your nervous system and physiology influence your feelings, thoughts, and behaviors.

Harkening back to the discussion about brain, gut, metabolism, and blood sugar: understanding, planning, programming, and gradually modifying your self-control takes knowledge and accommodation to how your individual body and brain operate. Exercising progressively informed choices in food selection will change your habits, self-image, ease of adopting better habits, and ultimately your body size.

Whereas the bottom line determinants of weight and appetite are based upon the foods we eat and how our metabolism functions (genetic influences included), controlling stress and modulating self-regulation heavily affect our abilities to do so on a sustained basis. Regular consumption of unhealthy food breeds fat, illness, and much discomfort. But even armed with knowledge about how to eat healthier, our emotions, traumas, brain dysregulation, and self-defeating beliefs easily interfere with executing our will and intention for self-improvement. This is why I have devoted so much of my professional efforts toward helping people gain control of mind, body, stress, and the self-indulgences that lead to escape and self-medication to deter feelings of anxiety and deprivation.

Becoming friends with food and eating encompasses the following truths:

- Reduced obsessive thinking and preoccupation with food is relative, but consider that constantly reviewing what you will eat next elevates food and eating to an unfavorable echelon.

- Food and eating should be enjoyable, not fraught with unmanageable restrictions, minute counting of ingredients or calories, or harsh internal dialogue.

- Healthy anticipation of eating meals or snacks is part of life's pleasure. This gets easier when blood sugar is regulated and stress does not yank us into impulsive capitulation to relieve anxiety or lower blood sugar.

- You can *gradually* learn to like, prefer, and yearn for foods that are healthier for you—just as you can grow to appreciate and admire qualities in someone else that previously you disdained. Tastes can change. It takes practice and new habits.

- Even with a plan and program to gradually eat healthier, indulgences and relapses are part of being human. Periodic reversions to indulgences are not signs of failure. They can help stave off feelings of deprivation or suffering. And it is often the case that after eating more healthfully, binges or regressions will not satisfy in the same way they did previously. Some people follow the 90–10 or 80–20 "rule"—healthy adherence most of the time with some allowance for going "off the food wagon." Of course, those with food allergies, sensitivities, or other health issues must be cognizant and careful in this regard.

- From an evolutionary perspective, our bodies and motivations orient toward eating more because food used to be scarcer in human history. Food is now abundant in much of the world, but our bodies are still programmed to store up calories in order to avoid scarcity or starvation. Our desire and motivation to eat beyond immediate hunger is biologically founded. Though some natural tendencies need to be diverted and controlled, this does not necessitate self-loathing or punishment.

- The dependability factor in friendship can also be applied to the way we relate to food and our bodies. We want and expect our bodies to serve us reliably, to function routinely and without constant pain or discomfort. In turn, we must treat our bodies with diligent care and attention, supplying our systems with the fuel and ingredients needed to flourish. You wouldn't knowingly serve your friends meals that are spoiled or bad for them. Treat yourself with similar care and respect.

• Friendship with your body implies that you like doing things together—that is, your mind, motivation, and intention should become compatible with what your body can enjoy and tolerate. This plays out in digestion, exercise, rest and relaxation, and social and work activities. Though we all must fulfill tasks and obligations we might prefer to avoid, treating our bodies with spartan discipline does not encourage friendship or feeling at ease. You wouldn't insist that a friend run more minutes than they can tolerate, so why incur harsh standards upon yourself?

Variations in Other Bodies

I have always loved dogs. I take my dog to the park regularly. This routine provides me with ready observation of many different types of dogs. Over the last few centuries, humans have purposefully crossbred dogs to create newer breeds. The combination of natural selection and human intervention has produced a wide assortment of canine appearances and bodies.

People have different preferences in the dogs they choose as pets and in their views and biases about the attractiveness, temperaments, and desirability of various dogs. With the wide and stark variation in the way dogs look, how they move, and how much they weigh, we see fat dogs, skinny dogs, large, medium, and small ones, very furry and less furry, squat and lithe, etc. But I feel fairly confident that dogs don't berate themselves or each other over how they look. They just are who they are and live with it.

Our judgments—for whatever they are worth—are not reflected self-consciously in how dogs see themselves and other dogs. If only a bit of this natural acceptance would rub off on humans! God and nature evolved different shapes, sizes, and appearances in mammals and other life forms. Even though many of us (and our dogs) may need to modify eating habits for our health, this is no reason to eschew our nature or how we look.

Surely, people are sensitive to body-shaming in ways that probably escape dogs. This is unfortunate and hurtful. But with adequate ego strength, increasing confidence, and a secure self-acceptance, we can recognize that the negativity and slurs from others simply reveal their own insecurity and judgmental insensitivity. We don't have to own or internalize what others say when they announce their criticisms.

Different Sizes for Comfort

When my children were teenagers, we went to Hawaii. My older son led me to a clothing store that offered the latest fashions. He wanted to buy some clothes to "fit in" in the stylish sense.

While he was shopping, I tried on some shorts in the largest size the store had available: XXX-large. At the time, I was about a hundred pounds heavier than I am now. Though accustomed to finding that in many brands and styles, even the largest sizes fit me tightly and were unbecoming, I was shocked to discover that in this particular store, the largest XXX-large shorts would not even fit above my thighs. Oh, how mortified and embarrassed I was! This was not just a matter of being overweight; this store and its brands catered to younger and very different body types. I felt like a whale in a kiddie pool!

Being overweight brings unpleasant reminders and difficult adjustments. Airplane seats are a challenge, finding flattering and fitting clothing is hard, and even much of the furniture designed for smaller bodies can frustrate larger people fraught with limited selection, higher prices, and much self-castigation.

Different body types and sizes are a reality, partly through nature's diversity and partly through the swelling epidemic of obesity. I emphasize: even as you may be trying to reduce your size, don't add pointless and self-denigration to your self-image and dignity.

Clearly, in this struggle, you are not alone.

Path to Self-Regulation, Acceptance, and Friendship

We ought to like ourselves as much as we can, based on natural compassion, realistic self-assessment, and a blending of structured self-improvement habits, and reasonable goals and achievable standards. I can't provide a specific prescription that works for every person, but I can recommend that you examine and reflect upon your standards in judging and relating to others as well as yourself. Though some people are uncannily too critical of others while blind to their own shortcomings, most people judge and criticize themselves way too harshly.

What people think up for themselves, their worst enemies wouldn't wish upon them. Does this phrase resonate with you? Have you been too hard on yourself? Do you yield to negative comparisons that diminish your own value and integrity?

Perhaps it's time to seek and espouse more kindness toward than gustatory indulgence for yourself. This you do deserve!

Attitude, effort, planning, proper evaluation, knowledge, and practice work together to form and reinforce better habits and more satisfying and tangible results.

Foster an Enduring Friendship

Building and sustaining a friendship with yourself, your body, and with food and eating takes a confluence of emotional, psychological, and neurological healing along with gradual changes in habits and physiological adaptation and regulation.

We all need to set reasonable goals that encourage consistent progress toward cumulative short-term and longer-term success. Quick weight-loss methods don't last, and you've probably found that out. Pounding at the gym for several hours may also overdo it and is not likely to yield the results you want.

Individual strategies vary, but most people can benefit from some medical advice and/or supervision, research and/or coaching on food selection, peer support, and perhaps professional intervention to treat the brain and physiology issues that obstruct. Just as most friendships require adjustment, accommodations, and some sacrifices, treating yourself well and respectfully will lead you to altering maladaptive patterns of rewards and indulgences. For the most promising success, this should be done over time without sudden or spartan restrictions. The idea is to avoid feelings of deprivation or suffering as you reestablish your relationship with yourself and food. You really can become friends!

As you get better at regulating blood sugar, your improving control over appetite will allow you to plan meals and snacks and become satisfied with healthier foods and less volume. With deliberate intention and practice, you can find ways to relieve stress other than eating.

Consider the importance of healing your traumas and developing methods of releasing negative emotions. Enslavement to food takes terrible tolls beyond detriments to physical health. Food obsessions distract from the wide array of pleasures, necessities, and focus that provide meaningful and lasting rewards.

What your parents did and however they fed you pales in relevance to what you eat now (and how it may play havoc with your brain and body). Success derives from how you adjust your attitudes and self-acceptance; getting rid of the traumas that shackle you to self-hate, self-medicating, and escape; and your implementation of modern, effective methods for developing self-control of your mind and body.

Toward those we love and treat with respect, we express our appreciation, ask for help, compromise our needs and expectations, and strike an acceptable balance between giving and getting. We must strive to achieve similar functional and satisfying objectives in becoming better friends with ourselves and with the good food that nourishes and sustains us.

I want you to feel good about yourself! God created you with special interests in mind. There is no one exactly like you, and you need not try to be like someone else. Follow healthy principles, do your best, and work on accepting yourself. Cultivate inner beauty, even as you strive to slim down and gain more self-control. More important than achieving a certain weight or size is appreciating yourself, loving others, and divesting yourself of unrealistic standards and perceived imperfections.

If you are interested in guidance, mentoring, treatment, or just encouragement, feel free to contact me. I am interested in *you*.

Other Reading on Diet and Nutrition

Campbell, PhD, T. Colin and Thomas M. Campbell II, MD. *The China Study: Revised and Expanded Edition.* The Most Comprehensive Study of Nutrition Ever Conducted and the Startling Implications for Diet, Weight Loss, and Long-Term Health. BenBella Books, 2016.

Greger, MD, FACLM. Michael. *How Not to Diet: The Groundbreaking Science of Healthy, Permanent Weight Loss.* Flatiron Books, 2019.

Kessler, MD, David. *The End of Overeating: Taking Control of the Insatiable American Appetite.* Simon and Shuster, 2009.

Kessler, MD, David. *Fast Carbs, Slow Carbs: The Simple Truth About Food, Weight, and Disease. Harper.* Audio, 2020.

Moss, Michael. *Salt Sugar Fat: How the Food Giants Hooked Us.* Random House, 2013.

Moss, Michael. *Hooked: Food, Free Will, and How the Food Giants Exploit Our Addictions.* Random House, 2021.

Acknowledgments

Along my own journey to better health, weight loss, self-control, and satisfaction, I sought the medical expertise of truly outstanding physicians. I profoundly thank cardiologist David Kurzrock, MD, whose diagnosis and care for my advanced heart disease saved my life. I am also indebted to family physician Arkady Gendelman, MD, whose meticulous care and follow-up over the years provided me with knowledge, direction, medical care, and encouragement. Both of these physicians answered my questions patiently and repeatedly with the most current medical knowledge. They helped me restore my metabolism to more normal and healthy functioning. As a result, I am healthier, thinner, more energetic, and living with significantly less pain and worry about my health.

I thank Marly Cornell, who edited this book and two of my previous books. She has meticulously refined my message and style with tactful and direct suggestions and critiques. She's managed to improve my writing without eroding my confidence or motivation. I am so grateful for her help and collaboration.

My thanks also to the Mayfly Design team, Julie, Ryan, and staff, for your talent and gracious assistance with this publication.

Mark Steinberg PhD
September 2024

153

About the Author

Dr. Mark Steinberg is a licensed psychologist with expertise in clinical, educational, and neuropsychology. Throughout a practice spanning four decades, Dr. Steinberg has administered more than 100,000 evaluation and treatment procedures, treating children, adolescents, and adults. He offers a range of services dealing with attention and mood disorders, behavior problems, family and communication issues, developmental disabilities, educational and learning problems, parenting challenges, habit change, addictions, and neurological disorders (including headaches, seizures, and sleep disorders).

By blending the latest technological advances with traditional and scientific methods, Dr. Steinberg improves functioning and eliminates problems that have often persisted for years. He is well-known for his pioneering work with EEG neurofeedback and voice technology, treatment that eliminates negative emotions in minutes.

Widely consulted as a medical expert, and the winner of local and statewide awards, Dr. Steinberg has made many appearances on local and national television, offering psychological expertise on topics pertaining to health, behavior, and how to live a more satisfying and productive life.

Dr. Steinberg offers individual services, seminars, and trainings.
For more information:
Call (**408**) **356-1002**
Visit **www.marksteinberg.com**

Other Publications by Mark Steinberg, PhD

Reality Reports: Essays on Mental, Emotional, Spiritual, and Social Issues in the Twenty-First Century. https://marksteinberg.com/webpages/reality -reports.jsp

Overcome Anxiety: Break Free From Fear, Worry, Trauma, and Negative Thinking (2023)

Life Control: Take Charge and Get Ahead (2023)

When God Takes Away: Living with Loss and Surrender (2016)

Confessions of a Maverick Mind: A Psychologist Shares Stories and Adventures, Essays and Articles, and Poems and Songs (2014)

Living Intact: Challenge and Choice in Tough Times (2012)

Staying Madly in Love with Your Spouse: Guide to a Happier Marriage; and *Living Intact: Challenge and Choice in Tough Times.* (2012)

ADD: *The 20-Hour Solution*, with Siegfried Othmer, PhD (2004)